"How I Lost 45 lbs in 3 Months Eating a Traditional American Breakfast – And How You Can, Too"

CHRIS MIQUEL & JASON PARSONS

Copyright © 2018 Wholly Fit Marketing All rights reserved. No part of this publication may be reproduced, distribute, or transmitted in any form or by any means, including photocopying, recording, or other electronic or mechanical methods, without the prior written permission of the publisher, except in the case of brief quotations embodied in reviews and certain other non-commercial uses permitted by copyright law.

ISBN: 978-1-9830-9293-0

DEDICATION

I would like to dedicate this book to the following people:

To my father, Dr. Roberto Jorge Miquel, who I lost at a very young age. He is a catalyst for my lifestyle change.

To my mother, Maria Luisa Miquel, for allowing me to be myself even when I was lost and for trusting in me that I would figure it all out.

To my two amazing kids, Victoria and Antonio, the reasons I embarked on this journey of living a fitter, healthier, and happier life. I will do everything in my power to be around for you two as long as I can.

To my beautiful wife, Karla, for supporting me through the entire process and all the years of entrepreneurship. She has trusted me throughout the process and loved me unconditionally through all the ups and downs.

And to all the fakers who come up with gimmicky diets and take advantage of consumers who spend their hard-earned dollars for something that will not work in the long run. You are the reason so many people fail, and I want to expose the truth and educate consumers on how to properly eat any type of food.

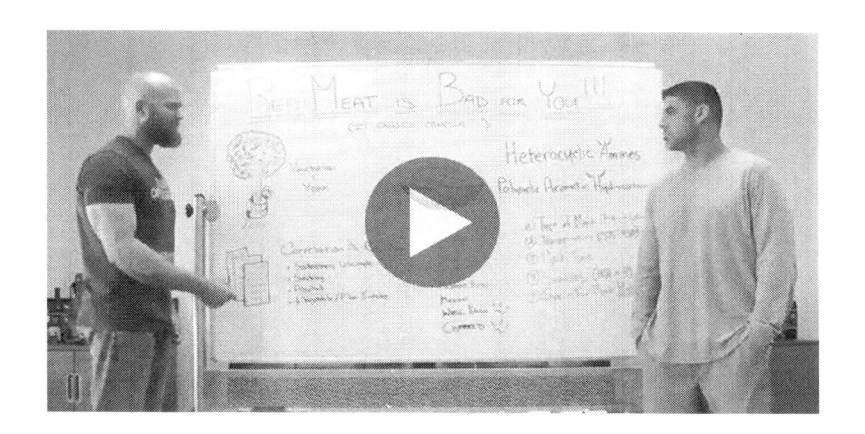

FACT OR FICTION?

Every Friday the Professor and I launch a new video where we expose the truth about many of the most common fitness myths.

TO WATCH THESE EPISODES GO TO:

http://overeasylife.com/videos

FOLLOW ME

@THEOVEREASYLIFE

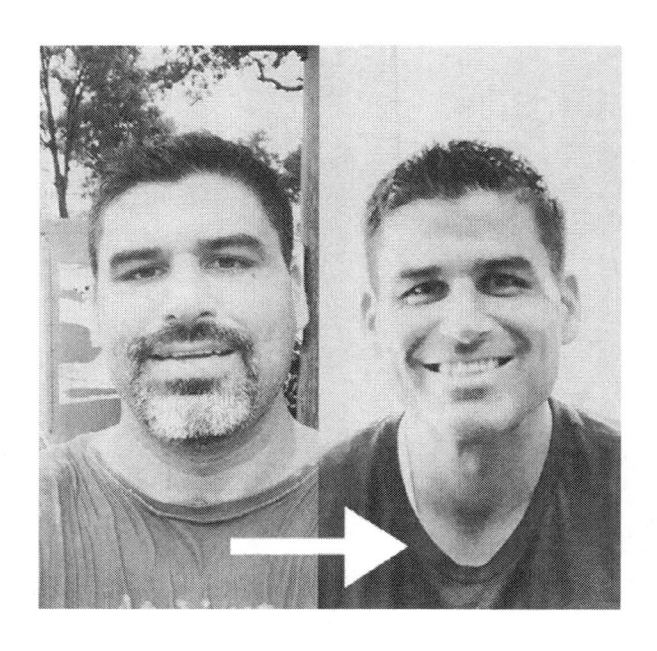

And be part of my journey of living a fitter, healthier, and happier life.

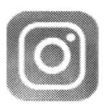

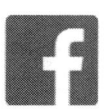

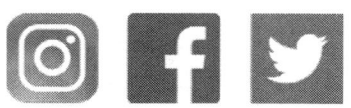

FOREWORD

I am often called a "big child" by my wife, despite the 40-plus times I have ridden this big rock we call Earth around the Sun. I suppose it is due to my never-ending curiosity to learn about the world around me. On a daily basis, I find myself curious about the world around me, filling my head with questions: "Who?" "How?" "Why?" "When?", which is why I prefer to think of myself as a lifelong student as opposed to being a "big child," but you won't find me arguing with my wife about it because I don't want to get put on another time-out.

I have enjoyed a long career as a personal trainer working with professional athletes to improve their mile time, young children who want to be better at basketball, stay-at-home parents who suffer from low-back pain, and cute little old ladies who just want to keep up with their doggies when they go for a walk. Across the board, the clients who ended up getting the best results were those who had the same childish curiosity that I exhibit on a daily basis. This is what I believe is the defining characteristic that has helped Chris Miquel to achieve so much success with his health transformation in such a short period of time: curiosity. Chris and I have developed a great relationship over the years we have worked together, due in part to our kindred spirit when it comes to wanting to learn. Chris is a computer wizard, and he has mentored and empowered me to better leverage technology in my fitness career so that I might spread the word of health and fitness to an even greater audience than I ever thought possible. On the other side of the coin, Chris has constantly peppered me with questions and skepticism during the time we have spent working on his fitness goals. And due to his intensive note-taking and ironclad memory, he has managed to achieve incredible results not only with his own body but now also with this book, *The Overeasy Life*. Chris is paying forward the insight and understanding about nutrition and the human body that he extracted from me during our time working as trainer and client.

In my time as a personal trainer, I have seen many of my clients achieve great results, and some were so inspired by their results that they even went on to become personal trainers themselves. In all these years, however, I have never had a client take such diligent notes and ask so many probative questions that they were able to actually write a book like Chris has here. When Chris approached me with the idea of sharing all that he has learned and used to achieve his own health and fitness goals, I was at first very skeptical that he would be able to do justice to the long talks we shared on the wide array of topics we had covered. Imagine my surprise when he presented me with the first rough draft of this book.

Chris is not only conveying all the relevant scientific concepts that need to be understood and followed to ensure the best fat loss results possible, but he does it in a manner that I typically find quite challenging. He speaks in a language everyone can embrace: personal experience. You see, I have never been overweight, nor have I struggled with proper nutrition. Eating healthy foods and staying in good shape have always just been a normal part of my life, so there have been many conversations with my clients that just didn't seem to "connect" as I was speaking from a place of scientific understanding more so than from experience. This is where Chris has me beat: he understands the science of how to lose weight AND has the experience of having actually dropped dozens of pounds of fat off his very own body.

This book is truly the embodiment of the phrase "The student becomes the master" as Chris has taken all the scientific knowledge that I shared with him, coupled it with his own real-world experience in dropping over 45 pounds of fat in just 3 months, and wrapped it up with great storytelling into this amazing book. While he might call me "The Professor" due to my extreme scientific nerdiness, it is Chris who has established himself as the authority on how to change your life through proper nutrition with this great book you are about to read. With *The Overeasy Life*, the student truly can become the master.

- Jason M Parsons, CSCS,
CPT - *ACE, ISSA, NASM, ACSM, NSCA, NESTA*
April 2018

CONTENTS

INTRODUCTION   1

Section 1:
MY STORY

    THE PROFESSOR AND I   17

Section 2:
FOODS THAT ARE OPTIMAL TO HELP LOSE FAT AND BOOST ENERGY!

    CHOLESTEROL AND FATS ARE YOUR FRIENDS
                                                  26
    CARBOHYDRATES TO THE RESCUE   31
    RESISTANT STARCHES   34
    PROTEIN AND YOU   37
    HI. MY NAME IS CHRIS, AND I AM ADDICTED TO CAFFEINE.   41
    PLANNING OUT YOUR FOOD   44
    IN SUMMARY   49

Section 3:

WHEN SHOULD YOU EAT TO MAXIMIZE RESULTS?   54

    INTERMITTENT FASTING   57
    SATIETY   63
    CARBOHYDRATES FOR FUEL   66
    COFFEE AS AN APPETITE SUPPRESSANT   68
    IN SUMMARY   69

Section 4:
HOW MUCH FOOD SHOULD YOU BE CONSUMING TO ACHIEVE YOUR GOALS?

    CALORIES-IN   74
    BALANCED NUTRITION   79
    KEEPING RECORDS   83
    ACCOUNTABILITY   84
    IN SUMMARY   87

Section 5:
THE OVEREASY SYSTEM

    EAT TO LIVE   91
    EAT FOR PURPOSE   92
    LIVE TO EAT   92

Section 6:
THE LOWDOWN AND DIRTY TRICKS YOU CAN FOLLOW

Fast During the Work Week	96
Fast Before a Calorie Bomb	97
Switch to Vodka Soda	98
Eating That High-Fat Breakfast for Dinner	99
Keep Fruits and Vegetables at Home for Snacks	99
Fast on the Road	100
For the Love, Not for Boredom	100

Section 7:
INFLUENTIAL THOUGHTS FROM INFLUENTIAL PEOPLE

Section 8:
REVIEW, SAMPLE DAY, AND TAKING ACTION

SAMPLE DAY OF FOOD	123

Meal 1 - Cucumber Tomato Salad with Tuna and Almond Butter with Celery & Carrots 123

Meal 2 - BBQ Chicken Breast with Grilled Zucchini 124

Meal 3 - Breakfast Sandwich with Egg, Cheese, and Ham 124

SAMPLE MEAL WHEN BREAKING FAST 126

Option 1 - Bacon and Eggs 126

Option 2 - Steak and Eggs 127

TAKING ACTION 128

BONUS: 30 MINUTE OVEREASY EXERCISE PROGRAM 131

INTRODUCTION

Life is difficult enough as it is without your own food working against you. With so much going on in our busy lives every single day, the last thing you want to do is to try and wade through all the scientific studies out there in an attempt to figure out how you should be eating in order to regain control of your life. With so many competing "diets", trying to figure out which one is just right for you can get super confusing, and that is exactly why I created The Overeasy System.

I wanted to share with you the simple steps that I took to lose 45 lbs in just 3 months. Before I could publish this book, I needed to make sure that the research-backed nutrition information I put into it was as easy to digest (yes, that pun was intended) as possible so that anyone could take immediate action and start getting results from day 1.

As you proceed through this book and learn all about The Overeasy System, you will notice that I reference the science behind the concepts I speak to. More importantly, however, I "translate" all that science into actionable items anyone can make a part of their daily life.

Remember that knowledge is power, but if you don't have the ability to put it into action, the results will never come. That's why a big part of what makes The Overeasy System so powerful is that it's "easy."

Keeping the actionable concepts as simple as possible allows you to pick and choose which ones will work best in YOUR lifestyle, so you can start using them immediately. Possibly even more important, the simplicity of this system allows you to keep doing the "right things" for your goal instead of going through the typical yo-yo most people experience with diets that force them to eat things they don't like and jump through nutritional hoops that aren't sustainable.

The Overeasy System is the solution that will forever change your relationship with food for the better.

This book is broken up into four parts:

1. My Story - A background on how I learned all the easy-to-use concepts found in The Overeasy System.

2. What to Eat - Learn which foods are optimal to help lose fat and boost energy.

3. When to Eat - Determining when you should eat to maximize fat loss.

4. How Much to Eat - Understanding how much food you should be consuming to achieve your goals.

We will wrap it up with a complete review, including a sample day of meals and how to take action.

Each chapter ends with a summary of the most important concepts to make sure you have the key takeaways needed to start getting results from the very first day.

I not only want to make the information provided easy to understand, but I also want you to be able to take immediate action on the concepts you're about to learn.

Yes, I know "patience is a virtue," but in today's high-paced world, there is no good reason to wait one minute longer than necessary. Chapter by chapter, you will be accessing the very same concepts that helped me to lose 45 lbs in 3 months.

While my results might not be typical, the very same things I did to achieve these amazing fat loss results are now at your fingertips on the pages to come.

You will discover the OPTIMAL time to eat breakfast, which will help you blast away fat, pack on muscle, and regain the energy of your youth.

You will learn an incredibly simple change you can make with your current food intake that keeps you feeling fuller for longer and eliminates those pesky late-night cravings.

You will find out which of nature's "perfect foods" all the top nutritionists use to optimize results for just pennies a meal.

You will learn the EXACT amount of carbs you should be consuming to optimize fat-burning results, fuel your lifestyle, and keep those cravings under control.

You will discover how even people with the WORST eating habits can still get results that look photoshopped just by choosing this one type of delicious food you probably already have in the refrigerator.

You will learn which nutrient-dense foods help lower cholesterol and blood sugar, despite what doctors have been lying to you about for nearly 40 years!

You'll learn which DELICIOUS food you can put back on the menu, despite what all of the diet books and mommy bloggers are telling you.

Let's not waste any more time—it's time for you to see what makes The Overeasy System the solution to reaching your fat loss goals.

Section 1:

MY STORY

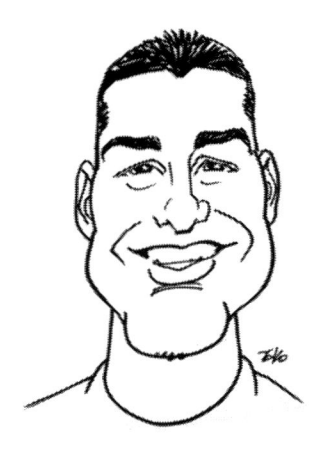

Hi! My name is Chris Miquel, and before I learned how to eat a high-fat breakfast for dinner, I was on a one-way road to the morgue.

Sounds pretty dramatic, doesn't it? Well, sadly, it is the truth.

My story starts way back in the 90s when I was in high school (Yeah, I am THAT old). At a time when everyone else was worried about fighting an outbreak of acne or trying to figure out which shirt color was going to make them one of the "cool kids," I was having trouble keeping my weight under control. It would go up and down randomly, and I just felt like my body was out of control. As if high school wasn't tough enough already, I was stuck in a constant battle with how my clothes fit, and I was scared to death about changing clothes in front of the other guys in the locker room.

Fast-forward to my 38th birthday. I was now running my own business, married to my best friend, and blessed with two amazing kids... oh, and I was the heaviest I've ever been in my life. Apparently, even though I was now an adult, I still hadn't figured out how to control my own body, and boy was it taking its toll on my overall health and wellbeing.

I mean, it's not like I am super lazy or anything—I am actually a pretty active guy who likes to run a few times a week, and I even hit the gym pretty regularly. So, how is it that I was still gaining weight? Yes, I know, the "average American" is a little more, how shall I put it, "robust" than they used to be, but that doesn't mean I was happy being average. The extra weight meant I had to buy bigger and bigger clothes, and even though I was no longer in high school, my extra weight still made me self-conscious about how I looked and what others thought of me.

Yeah, it kinda sucked worrying if other people were judging me based on how I looked. I wasn't too happy about that.

But, wait, there's more!

I visited my doctor for an annual check-up, and he told me that my cholesterol was through the roof. Great! He prescribed me cholesterol medication to try and lower it, and let me tell you how bad the side effects of cholesterol medication suck. Every time I took the medication, I felt like I had butterflies in my stomach for the entire day. I'd only feel normal for the first few minutes after I woke up, and then I'd start getting that weird feeling again. You know, that nervous feeling where the bottom of your stomach feels like it's in your throat. Now, imagine feeling like that all day long.
It seems that the medication was making me anxious, which would cause shortness of breath and eventually lead to a panic attack. The medication was driving me crazy, and I knew I couldn't keep going in that direction.

Oh, did I forget to mention how taking the cholesterol medication KILLED my sex drive? Yeah, neither me nor my wife were too pumped about that side effect. I had enough of these crappy side effects and decided to stop taking the medication, at a detriment to my overall health.

NOW, I was the fattest I've ever been and suffering from high cholesterol. Talk about a bad combo!

It was at this point that I had an aha moment, and I knew it was time for me to make a change if I wanted to be there for my kids when they were growing up.

When I was younger, being overweight was more of a nuisance, but now that it was impacting my health and I had other people in my life who depended on me, I had to make a change for their benefit.

Just in case my story isn't already tugging hard enough at your heartstrings, let me share one more detail with you about why I finally decided it was time to make a change.

Sadly, I know firsthand what it feels like to lose a parent as I lost my father in my senior year of high school from a heart attack. It was sudden and devastating for me and my entire family, and that pain of loss is a major motivator for me today to be as healthy as possible for my own children. It pains me deeply when I see others interacting with their fathers as I never got to enjoy our time together as adults. And I'd be damned if I was going to let my two little angels be put in a situation like that if I had any say in it.

Truth be told, it's not like I waited all these years to try and change how my body looked and felt. I've done the same thing as everyone else. I tried more diets than I care to admit (we are talking double digits here!). Juicing, fasting, South Beach Diet, Atkins, Zone Diet, and more. I've got so many stupid diet books sitting around my house that it looks like I am trying to open my own Barnes & Noble. None of these diets ever worked for me. Sure, I might lose a couple pounds in the first few days, but I usually hated the foods I had to eat, and I just couldn't sustain the diets for very long and simply gave up.

Heck, I even took the EXTREME route of cutting out all alcohol for an entire month (crazy, right?), and after 30 days of suffering, I had found that I didn't lose a single pound. What gives?

Now, I'm not a quitter, but I just wasn't finding a diet that fit me as an individual. It felt like every diet book I bought was trying to force me to conform to eating meals I didn't really enjoy or that were so different from what the rest of my family was eating. They really made me feel like a weird outcast who was force-feeding himself "twigs and berries" like it was some kind of punishment. My heart wasn't into it, so I didn't stick with these diets, and the results never came.

To me, being overweight and wanting to make a change seemed like such a giant mountain to climb that I always talked myself out of following through. I had the same list of worries as everyone else about why I just couldn't get results with a new diet:

"I won't be able to eat the foods I like...and that SUCKS!"

"I have to stop drinking adult beverages (frosty, cold beer), and that is going to RUIN my football tailgating—a pretty important part of my life (Go Dolphins!)."

"I have to cut out all carbs from my meals, and we all know THAT isn't going to happen because carbs taste awesome!"

"I've tried so many diets before, and they didn't work. Why would a new one be any different?"

On one hand, I was super bummed out about the prospect of even trying another diet, but on the other hand, I had my amazing wife and my two beautiful kids, who deserved to have me around for as long as possible. I felt like I was stuck between a rock and a hard place (that served Cinnabons). I had to do something, but what?

This is where the gym comes in. No, not because I found some killer workout plan that could magically erase my crappy eating habits, but rather because I found someone who helped change my perspective on food.

For the last few years, I had been going to the gym that is right downstairs from my work office. It is super convenient, and I know if I had to drive even one extra mile, I would probably talk myself out of it after a long day of arguing with my computer. I was a "regular" at the gym and knew quite a few people that worked out at the same time as I did. What I hadn't done (in hindsight, I feel silly for not thinking of this) was ask the people I interacted with every day what they were doing to get the great results they were achieving.

Week after week, I had watched from the relative safety of my trusty treadmill as person after person shed off excess body fat seemingly right before my very eyes. It was both maddening and inspiring, and one day I had had enough. In the middle of one of my daily treadmill sessions, I popped out my headphones and asked Justin on the treadmill next to me what was his "secret" for losing all the weight I had noticed he was shedding over the past few months.

Justin made a joke about me being a stalker, and then, with a casual laugh, he said he had gotten some great advice from a personal trainer that he had worked with at the gym, and it had changed how he looked at food. Curious, I asked if he had recommended he follow some specific new diet that I may not have heard of. With a smile on his face, he said no. He had simply given him some insight into what was REALLY going on with the foods he was already eating. He was then able to change the quantity and timing of his food intake to get the results he was looking for. He said the secret to his results came down to one basic thing: he started eating a high-fat breakfast for dinner, and the pounds just fell off.

Needless to say, I was super skeptical, and after chatting with Justin a little more, I asked him which trainer he had talked to. He pointed across the gym floor at a big bald guy named Jason, who he referred to as "The Professor." Apparently, Jason was some kind of super nutrition nerd who read research studies for entertainment and loved to chew your ear off about the science behind weight loss. Justin said that Jason had helped him to better understand the "real truth" about how food affects you, so that he could make better choices on his own.

I thanked Justin for sharing what had worked for him, and at that moment, I made up my mind to reach out to him and ask for some help. I had tried everything on my own and just wasn't getting the job done. Now, I owed it to myself and my family to take a chance and seek out professional help to change my life for the better.

What did I have to lose?

I'll tell you what I had to lose...: about 50 pounds!

Fast-forward through many hours of personal training sessions with Jason, and here I am today, with a new appreciation for what and how I eat foods and, more importantly, an optimistic outlook on achieving the weight loss and overall health goals I have for myself. This fitness and nutrition guru had totally changed my mindset on the everyday foods I already had in my house and on how I could use them to my weight-loss advantage instead of letting them pack on even more unwanted pounds.

Imagine my surprise when I learned that by simply changing how much and what time I ate certain foods that I already loved to eat, I could not only lose the weight I had so desperately wanted to get rid of, but I could also boost my overall energy and begin to return my elevated cholesterol levels to normal. I wouldn't believe it myself if I hadn't experienced it firsthand.

Steak and eggs for dinner? Ribs and a couple frosty beers with my buddies at the tailgate party? Foods that tasted great and were already in my refrigerator and pantry? Yeah, I was just as shocked as you are right now, but let me tell you what: it works.

I was finally able to stick to a food plan that I made for myself and enjoy the things I ate. I wasn't trying to force down an egg white omelette (gross!)

or plain boiled chicken breasts (even grosser!), and, surprisingly enough, I didn't have to pretend to enjoy eating "twigs and berries" anymore. Rather, I got to eat the foods I loved as the pounds started to melt off.

Who would have thought this was possible?

OK, OK, I know, "Let's get to the good stuff, Chris! Tell us what the heck you were eating so we can try it too!" Alright, I will walk you through all of the great information I learned from Jason (minus the thousands of dollars I wisely invested with him). I felt it was important that I share my story first so you could see I am just a regular guy like many of you out there. And the reality is, I didn't do anything "magical" to get the great results I have achieved. Instead I learned how to make some simple decisions every day to have my food work FOR me instead of AGAINST me.

The information I learned was profound enough to change my entire thinking about food, but not so specific that it was meant for only me. Jason has helped change the lives of thousands of people from all walks of life with this same information:

- Single moms who are facing significant time restrictions between their jobs and their children.

- Busy executives who have great business success but still haven't figured out how to control their health through proper food intake.

- Dads just like me who want to be around for their kids as long as possible.

- Older adults who are suffering the negative effects of diabetes or high blood pressure.

All these people and more have found immense benefit from learning the information I am about to share with you. The truth of the matter is that the old fishing adage really is true:

"Give a man a fish and he eats for a day; teach a man HOW to fish and he will eat for a lifetime."

Bouncing from fancy diet to fancy diet was never going to work for me as I wasn't really learning how to eat properly... until I spent some time learning from Jason. He actually taught me "how to fish," and now I can make my own nutritional decisions that get me the results I want, instead of blindly following a premade diet that forces me to eliminate some random "bad" food.

Are you ready to have your mind blown?

Do you want to know how eating steak and eggs for dinner can help you to lose more weight than you ever thought possible?

Buckle up because this might be a bumpy ride, my friend.

THE PROFESSOR AND I

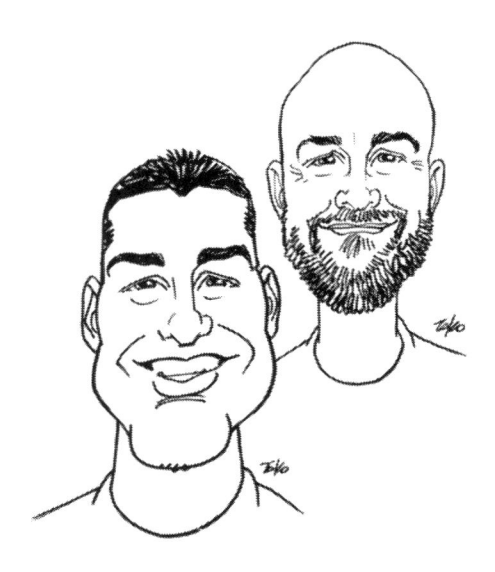

As it turns out, a large part of why I gained so much excess weight over my life is that the foods I was eating were SAD.

No, I don't mean the foods were depressed (although the weight I gained did kinda make me frown a little..). Rather, the things I always ate were part of the Standard American Diet, aka SAD[1].

I was overeating highly processed foods that have excessive amounts of sugar like pasta, soda, chips, and cookies, and at the same time I was avoiding foods that have saturated fats like whole eggs, butter, and rib eye steaks (yum!).

Why was I doing this?

I would love to tell you it was based in sound logic and science, but honestly I LOVE sweets and things with lots of sugar in them because, well, they taste good!

Also, I tended to avoid foods higher in saturated fats because for my entire life I had been told that foods that were high in saturated fat and cholesterol were the devil and would cause heart disease. And after what happened with my own father, I wanted to steer clear of anything that messed with my heart.

Who would have thought that in an effort to avoid eating things that would negatively affect my heart health, I was actually setting myself up for failure.

---

[1] Carrera-Bastos, Pedro; Fontes; O'Keefe; Lindeberg; Cordain (March 2011). "The western diet and lifestyle and diseases of civilization"

On one of the very first sessions working with The Professor, we sat at a desk for an entire hour and talked about my food habits, and boy was it eye-opening. Jason told me to walk him through everything I had eaten over the last three days, and as I started to share my (terrible) eating habits, he would stop me every once in a while and ask me things like

- "Why did you choose that specific food?"
- "Why did you eat that specific amount of food?"
- "Why did you eat at that specific time?"

As I am sure you can already guess, most of the time I didn't have a good answer, but rather I tended to say, "Because it tastes good" or "That's how much food was on my plate." To be honest, I was pretty shocked about just how little planning and thought actually went into my own food intake. I would basically choose what I ate based on three criteria:

1. Does it look good?
2. Does it taste good?
3. Is it convenient?

It was becoming all too apparent just from my answers to Jason's questions that I really had no plan at all as to what went into my mouth, and that surely wasn't a good thing.

After about 30 minutes of complete embarrassment from sharing my horrible dietary intake, Jason sat back in his chair and shared with me his observations about my day-to-day diet. I was sure he was going to blast me for all of the crap I had been consuming, but instead he smiled and told me not to worry and that I was going to be pleasantly surprised with how easy it would be to fix my diet.

I raised an eyebrow in suspicion and asked what he meant by "easy." Like I've told you before, I have tried all kinds of "diets" in the past, and MOST of them were a giant pain in the ass and required that I cut out entire food groups or that I eat bland foods I couldn't stand. I was justifiably skeptical about this "easy" claim Jason was making.

Boy, was I wrong.

It turns out that while I was NOT getting the results I wanted with my food (losing weight, keeping my cholesterol under control, and having more energy throughout the day), my diet didn't need a super complicated overhaul like I had assumed. Rather, all I needed to do was to better understand a few basic concepts that would empower me to make better food choices and get the results I had wanted all along.

Talk about a relief!

I was absolutely certain that this guy they called "The Professor" was going to give me a meal plan that was übercomplicated and required an advanced degree just to understand. In reality, Jason would spend the next few months with me carefully explaining these basic nutrition concepts in terms that I could understand and that made sense to me once he walked me through the science behind them. I've never been much of a science guy (I'm more of a computer geek), but thankfully Jason was able to translate all the complicated research studies that he used as references into the simple eating concepts that he helped make a part of my daily life.

To get my life back on track, I needed to wrap my head around the fact that my specific food choices had a profound effect on my results.

I know you're probably thinking right now:

"Duh, everybody knows that."

But hear me out because what I THOUGHT were the "right foods," well, it turns out I had been lied to all my life, just like you probably have, and those lies were keeping me from the results I so desperately wanted.

I had spent most of my life doing what I thought was "the right thing" with my food choices. I made sure most of the foods that I ate were starchy foods like whole grain breads and potatoes (chips and French fries, actually), and I avoided foods that had too much of the dreaded saturated fats and cholesterol because that is what every book and article had always taught me.

Heck, the dang food pyramid from the USDA[2] has always shown us that we are supposed to only have a tiny amount of fats in our diet (the top of the pyramid) and to consume the MOST of breads, cereals, and pasta (the bottom of the pyramid). It turns out I've been going about it all wrong as the food pyramid was a total lie.

---

[2] USDA MyPyramid

Section 2:

FOODS THAT ARE OPTIMAL TO HELP LOSE FAT AND BOOST ENERGY!

That very first sit-down with Jason turned out to be such an eye-opener that it left me feeling like my world had been turned upside down.

What I THOUGHT I had to do to eat right turned out to be the OPPOSITE of what was really going to get me the fat-burning, metabolism-building results I was looking for. After I had finished listing what I had eaten for the last few days, Jason said he was going to make me a very happy man with his very first food suggestion.

I raised an eyebrow and asked him to continue.

"Eggs. You're going to be able to eat a lot more eggs and not just the whites but the WHOLE egg."

This was both terrifying and eggciting (see what I did there?). Nearly my entire life, I had been taught that the fat and cholesterol in the egg yolk was a "heart attack waiting to happen," and with my family history, I wanted nothing to do with them. Now, this really sucks because I LOVE eating eggs—especially if they are accompanied with a nice juicy rib eye!

Yes, it's true, I am a HUGE fan of a good old country breakfast (steak and eggs, to be specific), even though most of my life I honestly believed it was going to be the death of me. I had mentioned this during my conversation with Jason, mumbling something about how I loved eating these kinds of food for breakfast but how I rarely did because I knew it was so bad for me. And now, here we are with Jason teasing me that I might be able to enjoy one of my favorite foods in the whole world? I wasn't going to have to try and choke down any more of those bland egg-white-only omelettes? Where do I sign up?

But, hold on a second here. What about all of that fat and cholesterol in the yolks? I thought that was bad for my heart health? I pushed back on Jason and told him what I had always heard on TV and read in magazines about the "evil" fats and cholesterol, and how I didn't want to risk messing up my already elevated cholesterol levels. I certainly didn't want to go back on that terrible cholesterol medication that was wrecking my life, so I was understandably skeptical of what Jason was saying.

That's when The Professor schooled me on the reality of how GOOD for you whole eggs really are[3].

Think about this: What is an egg?

It's all the materials needed to create life packed into a little stand-alone package. Proteins to build tissues like bone, muscle, skin, and feathers (in the case of chicken eggs)[4]. Fats to help create all of the structures of the nervous system, including the brain (that's right, the brain is the fattiest organ in the body, consisting of a minimum of 60% fat![5]). Carbohydrates/sugars to provide the needed energy for the newly formed life. On top of that, there are a multitude of vitamins, enzymes, and minerals all crammed into these perfect little sources of nutrition, most of which are in the yolk. You know, the part of the egg that for far too many years the "low-fat" and "anti-cholesterol" crowd has told you was bad for you. Have you ever suffered through a

---

[3] Takehiko Yamamoto, Lekh Raj Juneja, Hajime Hatta, Mujo Kim. 1996. ""Hen Eggs: Basic and Applied Science"
[4] Vliet, et al. 2017. ""Consumption of whole eggs promotes greater stimulation of postexercise muscle protein synthesis than consumption of isonitrogenous amounts of egg whites in young men"
[5] CY Chang, et al. 2009. "Essential fatty acids and human brain"

nasty egg white omelette? I wouldn't wish that on my enemies. Blah.

CHOLESTEROL AND FATS ARE YOUR FRIENDS

Jason explained to me that whole eggs and all of the fat and cholesterol contained in their yolks have gotten an incredibly bad rap for many years due to faulty logic: it was assumed that consuming cholesterol in your diet meant your blood-level cholesterol would go up, and you would have a higher risk of cardiovascular disease[6].

Once I found out that the TRUTH was that neither fat nor cholesterol was in fact a "bad guy," and that the majority of the "good stuff" in an egg was packed into that little yellow globe in the middle[7], well, that was when I started enjoying whole eggs again. I was freed from the manufactured guilt that should have never been there to begin with.

As if that wasn't good enough, whole eggs are one of the best dietary sources of choline, which is

[6] Richard, C., Cristall, L., Fleming, E., Lewis, E. D., Ricupero, M., Jacobs, R. L., & Field, C. J. 2017. "Impact of Egg Consumption on Cardiovascular Risk Factors in Individuals with Type 2 Diabetes and at Risk for Developing Diabetes: A Systematic Review of Randomized Nutritional Intervention Studies"
[7] Yang, et al. 2012. "An Egg-Enriched Diet Attenuates Plasma Lipids and Mediates Cholesterol Metabolism of High-Cholesterol Fed Rat"

essential for your metabolic and cardiovascular health and a nutrient that is lacking in many "no egg"-diets[8].

Yeah, you read that correctly: whole eggs can actually help keep your metabolism running on all cylinders and improves overall heart health.

Jason continued by telling me research shows that eggs—or more specifically, their yolks—are nutrient-dense superfoods that actually can improve the structure of your cholesterol molecules, leave your body's serum cholesterol levels mostly unchanged, and even help to improve the absorption of fat-soluble vitamins such as vitamins A, E, D, and K[9].

These studies even indicate that the consumption of three to four eggs per day is heart healthy (the OPPOSITE of what I had been told my entire life) and can help you prevent the accumulation of fat in your midsection[10].

---

[8] DiMarco, D., et al. 2017. "Intake of up to 3 Eggs/Day Increases HDL Cholesterol and Plasma Choline While Plasma Trimethylamine-N-oxide is Unchanged in a Healthy Population"
[9] Kim, Jung Eun, Mario G. Ferruzzi, and Wayne W. Campbell. 2016. "Egg Consumption Increases Vitamin E Absorption from Co-Consumed Raw Mixed Vegetables in Healthy Young Men"
[10] Kern Jr, Fred. 1991. "Normal plasma cholesterol in an 88-year-old man who eats 25 eggs a day: mechanisms of adaptation"

What's that phrase the younger crowd uses? Mind blown!

By making all these claims about how the cholesterol in egg yolks was not only NOT bad for me but could in fact be good for me, Jason really had me skeptical. As you already know, I had a major issue with elevated cholesterol levels, and I had even gone on one of those terrible prescription medications to try and lower my overall cholesterol levels.

As it turns out, dietary cholesterol intake just doesn't have as large of an impact on blood cholesterol for most individuals as was always assumed[11]. In general, eggs don't seem to have a negative effect on blood cholesterol measures, and a causative link between the consumption of dietary cholesterol and serum cholesterol does not exist[12].

SAY WHAT?!

Basically, eating foods high in cholesterol has no direct link to an increase in your blood cholesterol levels.

---

[11] Hopkins PN. 1992. "Effects of dietary cholesterol on serum cholesterol: a meta-analysis and review"
[12] Herron, Kristin L., et al. 2004. "High intake of cholesterol results in less atherogenic low-density lipoprotein particles in men and women independent of response classification"

Have you ever felt like you were living in the Matrix? Like everything around you was just a lie?

Yeah, that's pretty much what I thought after Jason broke down what was really going on with eggs, fats, and cholesterol.

I was honestly pretty upset that I had spent so many years cutting out higher-fat foods and replacing them with low-fat/no-fat options that tasted like cardboard and (as it turns out) weren't even helping to improve my cholesterol levels[13]. Truth be told, consuming a moderate amount of fat in your diet is actually preferred for most people, as long as you are able to keep your processed-sugar consumption under control—it's actually the combination of too much fat and too much sugar that causes a lot of the health problems for the average American[14].

I'll be honest with you: it took me a while not only to digest (pun intended) all this "world-altering" information I had learned from Jason but also to replace my old, "bad" habits of avoiding fats like they were the plague. I had so many years of

---

[13] Guay V., et al. 2012. "Effect of short-term low- and high-fat diets on low-density lipoprotein particle size in normolipidemic subjects"
[14] Enos RT, Davis JM, Velazquez KT, McClellan JL, Day SD, Carnevale KA, Murphy EA. 2012. "Influence of Dietary Saturated Fat Content on Adiposity, Macrophage Behavior, Inflammation, and Metabolism: Composition Matters"

programming from doctors, magazines, diet books, and nearly everyone around me telling me to avoid high-fat foods like they were going to smother me with a pillow in my sleep.

It was a shock at first, but after I was able to wrap my head around these basic concepts (saturated fat and cholesterol in my diet can be good for you), I began to get really eggcited (there it is again!) about eating breakfast again.

For too many years, I either ate bland oatmeal with egg whites for breakfast or skipped the meal altogether due to it being outright boring. It drove me crazy when I would travel for work, and everyone around me was enjoying a big, fluffy whole-egg omelet or a nice juicy steak and eggs for breakfast…and there I was, forcing down plain oatmeal with a fake smile on my face.

All that torture for nothing!

It looks like eggs are the "perfect food," and for the price, they definitely can't be beat… or can they?

Get it? Nevermind, we will continue.

CARBOHYDRATES TO THE RESCUE

So, after I finally got over the shock of how much misinformation I had been fed (yay, another pun!) over the years by doctors, magazines, infomercials, and even my so-called "friends" about fats and cholesterol, I realized I now had more questions than answers about my food intake.

What about all these claims that "carbs are bad for you" and the constant droning that sugar was the worst thing ever invented? Surely, there was some truth to this, right?

Yeah, not so much.

When posed this question, Jason simply smiled at me and reassured me that there was in fact no such thing as a bad food. I believe his actual words were something to the effect of "Do you think they commit crimes on the weekend or something?"

All joking aside, I honestly had believed for the longest time that sugar, especially white table sugar, was the worst thing you could possibly eat. As it turns out, not only is sugar NOT "bad" for you, but apparently sugar is the number one source of fuel that our bodies use on a daily basis, especially for the brain. Saying that sugar is bad for your body is kinda like saying that gas is bad for your car—it's pretty much the OPPOSITE of the truth.

Who would have known?

Carbohydrates—also known as sugars, oligosaccharides, and polysaccharides—are found in all types of fruits, vegetables, grains, legumes, tubers, and other foodstuffs. (What in the hell is a legume? Yeah, I didn't know either. The most popular legumes are peas, beans, chickpeas, lentils, and peanuts. And those tubers? They are things like potatoes, yams, sweet potatoes, and cassava known as yuca to us Hispanics). Without going into a super-sciency explanation, carbohydrates are essentially a form of stored energy that is created by plants when they use photosynthesis to convert the sun's energy into something more readily usable.

A very large percentage of the standard American diet is made up of processed carbohydrates in the form of simple sugars like glucose, sucrose, and fructose as they tend to taste good and are cheap to manufacture. If it's cheap and tastes good, it doesn't take a rocket scientist to figure out why they are so popular.

Overall, carbohydrates are the major source of energy for our bodies, so it should come as no surprise that we are "programmed" to seek out these types of foods and consume them when available. That's why our taste buds have evolved to sense sugars in the form of "sweet" tastes and also why, if given the chance, we will probably eat WAY more sugar than we actually need to survive.

This is the key bit of information to focus on with carbohydrates and sugar: too much is too much.

Carbs by themselves are NOT bad for you, but when consumed in excess, just like when ANYTHING is consumed in excess, they can and will cause weight gain. A recent study—the largest of its kind ever done—has shown that when it comes to losing weight there is no benefit to a low-carbohydrate diet as compared to a low-fat diet[15]. Ultimately, the most important factor is finding a diet that works best for the individual and allows them to stick with a reduced calorie intake long enough to see the results they are looking for.

Due to the natural desire for people to gobble up sweet-tasting foods whenever they are available, the average American will tend to overconsume carbs and gain unwanted extra weight, and that is why carbohydrates get such a bad name.

Jason explained to me long ago that when it comes to eating carbohydrate-laden foods like sweet

---

[15] Gardner CD, et al. 2018. "Effect of Low-Fat vs. Low-Carbohydrate Diet on 12-Month Weight Loss in Overweight Adults and the Association with Genotype Pattern or Insulin Secretion: The DIETFITS Randomized Clinical Trial"

potatoes, pasta, rice, beans, and breads, I was going to have to cut back a little (OK, a lot) as that was the food type I tended to overeat the most.

I am of Cuban descent and LOVE me some rice and beans, and as it turns out this may have contributed quite a bit to the extra pounds I have accumulated over the years—not because any of these foods are "bad" for me, but because I typically helped myself to GIANT portions and nearly always had a second helping. The recurring theme here is that I was overeating, and carbohydrate-based foods just happened to be my favorite thing to overeat.

For me, recognizing this and cutting back a little on the carbs and replacing them with some extra fats made an immediate difference in my weight loss as I was less hungry and just didn't want to have an extra serving of food anymore. Such a simple change that lead to the pounds starting to fall off.

RESISTANT STARCHES

One REALLY cool trick that I learned during all of this has to do with something called a "resistant starch."

As I said before, I am of Cuban descent, and foods high in starches (a type of carbohydrate) like rice, beans, and plantains have been a staple of my diet my entire life. So, I surely didn't want to have to give them up in order to drop the pounds needed to improve my health.

Apparently, these "resistant starches," which are found in the raw, uncooked forms of rice, beans and plantains, don't fully absorb in the small intestine, thereby essentially negating a large portion of their calories[16][17]. The problem is that, of course, NOBODY likes to eat raw, uncooked rice, beans, or plantains, and when cooked the resistant starches convert into regular starches, which your body will happily absorb.

Thankfully, as Jason explained, you don't have to eat these foods raw and uncooked to get the calorie-negating effects of the resistant starches. All you have to do is let these cooked foods cool down before you eat them.

Once cooled, most of the resistant starches that have been chemically modified into more absorbable forms of carbohydrates from the heat of cooking will revert to their original resistant starch

---

[16] Higgins JA. 2004. "Resistant starch: metabolic effects and potential health benefits"
[17] Bodinham CL, et al. 2010 " Acute ingestion of resistant starch reduces food intake in healthy adults"

form. Since they can't be absorbed very well in the small intestine, these resistant starches will pass down into the large intestine (colon), where intestinal bacteria ferment it, and short-chain fatty acids (SCFA) such as acetate, butyrate, and propionate, along with gases, are produced.

I know more crazy science stuff, but evidence suggests that all that fancy stuff (SCFAs) may benefit us in many ways[18][19].

For instance, they

- stimulate blood flow to the colon,
- increase nutrient circulation,
- inhibit the growth of pathogenic bacteria,
- help us absorb minerals, and
- help prevent us from absorbing toxic/carcinogenic compounds.

You get all these awesome benefits because you let the cooked rice, beans, and plantains cool down before eating them!

Crazy, right?

---

[18] Wolever TM, Spadafora P, Eshuis H. 1991. "Interaction between colonic acetate and propionate in humans"
[19] Grabitske HA & Slavin JL. 2009. "Gastrointestinal effects of low-digestible carbohydrates"

One thing I recommend NOT doing is having too much of this type of resistant starch all in one sitting. If you were paying attention above, you may have noticed where I said one of the byproducts of fermentation in your large intestine is gas. Unless you want to be really bloated and possibly make some new enemies in the elevator, you may want to slowly introduce this concept into your diet instead of going nuts with a couple huge sweet potatoes on the first try.

Trust me, I learned this lesson the hard way.

PROTEIN AND YOU

So, great. Fats, cholesterol, and carbohydrates aren't the bad guys, and in fact they can contribute to an overall heart-healthy and diabetic-friendly diet.

But, what about protein?

Everyone is always talking about protein like it's the greatest thing in the world, but in reality it is just another equally important piece of the nutrition puzzle.

Yes, we need protein to build the tissues of our body, not the least of which is that all-important muscle that powers us through our days and nights[20].

From a food-intake and meal-planning standpoint, protein can be used strategically to help maximize fat loss based on three very important factors:

1. Protein helps to spare muscle when in a caloric deficit[21]

2. Protein helps increase satiety[22]

3. Protein has a relatively high TEF (Thermic Effect of Food)[23]

Let me explain what each of these things means.

First off, maintaining a moderate to high amount of protein in your diet (30–40% of your total calories coming from protein) helps to minimize any muscle loss that typically occurs when someone is in a calorie deficit and trying to lose fat. While some

---

[20] Hulmi, Juha J., Christopher M. Lockwood, and Jeffrey R. Stout. 2010. "Review Effect of protein/essential amino acids and resistance training on skeletal muscle hypertrophy: A case for whey protein"
[21] Rittig, Nikolaj, et al. 2016. "Anabolic effects of leucine-rich whey protein, carbohydrate, and soy protein with and without β-hydroxy-β-methylbutyrate (HMB) during fasting-induced catabolism: A human randomized crossover trial"
[22] Makris AP, Borradaile KE, Oliver TL, Cassim NG, Rosenbaum DL, Boden GH, Homko CJ, Foster GD. 2011. "The individual and combined effects of glycemic index and protein on glycemic response, hunger, and energy intake"
[23] Kinabo, J. L., and J. V. G. A. Durnin. 1990. "Thermic effect of food in man: effect of meal composition, and energy content"

muscle loss is typically expected when a person is ingesting less food (measured in calories), that doesn't mean you have to relinquish more of your hard-earned muscle than necessary. Keeping a moderate to high level of protein intake is one way (resistance-training exercise is another) to make the majority of the weight you lose in this process come from fat as opposed to the "good stuff," your muscle.

Second, whenever you eat protein (and fats), regardless of the source (chicken, fish, eggs, dairy), that protein stimulates the production of cholecystokinin (CCK), a hormone that signals satiety, and inhibits the release of a hormone called ghrelin, which sends out the "I'm hungry" message. This leads to you feeling fuller for longer, and it can really help to prevent overeating[24].

Third, the actual chemical process of digesting and absorbing proteins requires the greatest amount of energy of all macronutrients[25].

The Thermic Effect of Food associated with eating protein basically "costs" about 20–35% of the total

---

[24] Yang D, Liu Z, Yang H, Jue Y. 2013. "Acute effects of high-protein versus normal-protein isocaloric meals on satiety and ghrelin"
[25] Quatela, Angelica, et al. 2016. "The Energy Content and Composition of Meals Consumed after an Overnight Fast and Their Effects on Diet Induced Thermogenesis: A Systematic Review, Meta-Analyses and Meta-Regressions"

available calories in the protein, which means you're essentially erasing those calories. The TEF for carbohydrates and fat is only 5–15%, less than half that of protein, so if a greater proportion of your food comes from protein sources, you are essentially consuming less total calories, and that change alone can have a profound effect on weight loss.

Let me explain that in simpler terms. You actually burn more calories when digesting protein than either fats or carbohydrates. If you consume 100 calories of protein, you will only have 65 to 80 calories of excess calories to fuel your body, while 100 calories of fats or carbs will leave you with 85 to 95 calories.

Something to note here: just as protein has a higher TEF, so do most "whole" foods as opposed to their processed versions. What I mean by that is that it requires more energy for your body to break down and digest the nutrients found in a whole apple than those found in apple juice. The same can be said of peanuts versus peanut butter, a steak versus ground beef, corn versus corn syrup, and lots of other foods that we consume regularly.

Choosing to consume "whole foods" that have been alive as recently as possible instead of their processed cousins is a great way to make your body work just a little bit harder to extract the nutrition.

Thinking about your food like this helps to eliminate some of the highly processed foods that are way too calorie dense, lacking in essential vitamins and enzymes, and devoid of real nutritional value. You also get the benefit of a higher TEF.

As you can see, these are some GREAT reasons to swap out some of your excess carbohydrates for some muscle-sparing, hunger-reducing proteins.

No, I am not saying carbs are bad, nor am i saying that protein is magical by any means, but again, now that you better understand how protein can be used strategically, you are better able to pick and choose your foods throughout the day to work FOR you instead of AGAINST you. Yeah, that's right, I'm helping to teach you how to get results on YOUR terms as opposed to just blindly following some fancy diet book that might not fit into your specific lifestyle.

Remember, "teach a man to fish" and he eats for a lifetime.

HI. MY NAME IS CHRIS, AND I AM ADDICTED TO CAFFEINE.

Sounds terrible, doesn't it? Well, it turns out that what I figured was one of my worst vices might actually be a pretty healthy habit after all. I typically go through 3 to 5 cups of coffee every day, and I'll tell you why it is a life saver for me.

Remember my two amazing kids I told you about in the beginning of this book?

I absolutely LOVE spending as much time with them as I can, so every day I get up early so that I can help get them up and ready for school before I head off to work myself. Just because I get up early every day to see my kids off to school and to hit the gym before work doesn't mean I'm a "morning person" by any stretch of the imagination.

Just like you, I need that "extra boost" of coffee first thing in the morning to help open my eyes fully so I can get on with my day. Honestly, I don't know what I would do without my "morning Joe", so it was a HUGE relief when Jason explained that I didn't have to cut back on my coffee, and he made me understand how coffee and caffeine (in controlled amounts) could actually be good for me!

Yay!

Jason explained hat caffeine helps to protect my brain functions against the wear and tear of stress (we all have a little too much of that in our lives!), plus it even helps to counteract the negative

42

aspects of the standard American diet that I had been consuming for so long[26].

Who knew caffeine was useful beyond its ability to wake me up?

Apparently, this increase in "energy" I was feeling every time I consumed some coffee (caffeine) wasn't just due to an improvement in mental alertness: there was an actual benefit to boosting my metabolism[27]!

I had always thought that consuming too much coffee was bad for me as it raised blood pressure, and because I was overweight to begin with, my doctors always told me to keep an eye on my blood pressure to avoid having to go on additional medications to keep it under control. You already know how I feel about medications, so it was a pleasant surprise to find out these rumors about coffee were totally untrue—I didn't have to cut back on my "addiction.[28][29]"

---

[26] Alzoubi KH, Abdul-Razzak KK, Khabour OF, Al-Tuweiq GM, Alzubi MA, Alkadhi KA. 2012. "Caffeine prevents cognitive impairment induced by chronic psychosocial stress and/or high fat-high carbohydrate diet"

[27] Astrup, A., et al. 1990. "Caffeine: a double-blind, placebo-controlled study of its thermogenic, metabolic, and cardiovascular effects in healthy volunteers"

[28] Mostofsky E, Rice MS, Levitan EB, Mittleman MA. 2012. "Habitual coffee consumption and risk of heart failure: a dose-response meta-analysis"

[29] Bøhn SK, Ward NC, Hodgson JM, Croft KD. 2012. "Effects of tea and coffee on cardiovascular disease risk"

PLANNING OUT YOUR FOOD

I suppose the "nice thing" here is that now that I have learned that there is no such thing as a "bad food" (e.g., carbs, fats, cholesterol, Twinkies…), I have been able to realign my entire way of thinking when it comes to planning my food throughout the day.

Where I once thought that eating carbs made me fat or at the very least kept me fat, I now know that carbs play a very important role in maintaining my energy levels throughout the work day as well as fueling my workouts. So, how do I plan my food out with this newfound information?

Let's walk through it.

First off, let's look at my work day.

I work in an office, and even though I have one of those fancy treadmill-desks that allows me to walk and type at the same time, the truth is I rarely use that feature. (It sure looks awesome whenever there are visitors, though, as it makes me look super-serious about my fitness.)

Basically, my work day is just a bunch of sitting at my desk, furiously moving my mouse around and typing stuff. Sounds fun, right? So, because MOST people out there also have similarly sedentary work environments[30] (not much physical activity), it's safe to say that the thought processes I use for planning out my food intake can be used by most of you as well.

Since I am NOT doing a whole lot of moving throughout the work day, I am using very little total energy (measured in calories), and what little I am using is being produced through fat metabolism.

Yeah, that's right, my body is a fat-burning machine while I am at work (yes, I am being sarcastic).

While the truth is that I actually am burning mostly fat while sitting at my desk, the real-world implication of this isn't all that exciting. I am burning so little total energy that it really doesn't matter where it comes from inside my body.

One of the most basic concepts I was taught by Jason is that your body uses two main energy sources: carbohydrates (glucose) and fat (yes, your body CAN use proteins and other sources, but it typically doesn't like to).

---

[30] Gordon-Larsen P, Nelson MC, Popkin BM. 2005. "Longitudinal physical activity and sedentary behavior trends: Adolescence to adulthood'

These energy sources (sugar and fat) are located all over the body—in your muscles, fat storage, bloodstream, liver, etc.. Your body picks and chooses which energy source it prefers and where to pull it from based on your activity intensity.

If you are doing a very low intensity activity (sitting at my desk), then your body will use fat (lipids) in the bloodstream plus oxygen for energy production as there is a low demand for energy. This is known as aerobic respiration.

When the demand for energy rises, the body begins to shift what it uses for energy production and where it gets it from. Sugar (glucose) becomes more and more in demand, and it typically is sourced first in the local tissues (muscles) followed by the bloodstream and then the liver[31].

Whew. That was a lot of science.

So, what does this have to do with planning out your food intake for the work day?

Basically, if a moderate to high level of physical activity isn't part of your typical work day (read: physical labor like construction), then in reality you probably do NOT need very much in the way of

---

[31] Romijn JA, Coyle EF, Sidossis LS, Gastaldelli A, Horowitz JF, Endert E, Wolfe RR. 1993. "Regulation of endogenous fat and carbohydrate metabolism in relation to exercise intensity and duration"

carbohydrates/sugar in your food intake as you have no real demand for it. The average American has a fairly sedentary lifestyle overall, including at work, and that typically means they don't have a real need for a lot of sugar in their diet.

Now, compare this to what the average American actually eats, and you'll begin to see why so many people are overweight and tend to have obesity-related diseases like hypertension and diabetes[32]. Sugar, especially the refined and concentrated version that we find in so many of our daily food and drink choices, is just not an "in-demand" macronutrient for the average American, so when they are over consuming sugar, it tends to get stored as extra body fat, and we all know how that works out.

Not so well.

Paying attention to what your life's demands are allows you to make wise food decisions, and in the context of what we are talking about here, you will be able to choose the types of foods that you consume so that they help you perform your best throughout the day, feel fuller for longer, and have the energy you need to feel great.

---

[32] Sullivan PW, Morrato EH, Ghushchyan V, Wyatt HR, Hill JO. 2005. "Obesity, inactivity, and the prevalence of diabetes and diabetes-related cardiovascular comorbidities in the U.S., 2000-2002"

If you have a lifestyle that requires you to be more active than the average person, you should plan to consume more carbohydrates/sugar as your body will need it and use it instead of storing it as extra body fat.

If you just aren't moving all that much on a day-to-day basis, it's a better idea for you to have a relatively lower amount of carbohydrate/sugar and maybe a little more fat in your diet as that is more in line with what your body uses for energy. Now, this is of course not an exact science, but the most important part of "learning how to fish" is firmly grasping the most important aspects of your nutritional intake, and "what you eat" is certainly one of them, especially based on what the demands of your life are.

Think about this: the typical off-the-shelf diet plan out there (Atkins, South Beach, Ketogenic) tends to try and force you and your unique lifestyle into their box, instead of allowing for total and free customization of your daily food intake like The Overeasy System teaches.

Yes, I know, it seems like there is way more "thinking" involved here than most people want to put into their nutritional intake. After all the other diets failed me due to their cookie-cutter structure, I was far more refreshed to take my results into my own hands by learning and practicing the simple concepts found here in The Overeasy System, as opposed to mindlessly eating the same things every day with little to no understanding of what works for my own body. I wasn't looking for a quick fix but a long-term solution. You know, "learning how to fish" as opposed to being given a fish.

IN SUMMARY

I've covered a lot of information here, so how do I actually apply all of this great stuff to my day-to-day eating? It's actually a lot simpler than you might think. Jason broke it down to me like this when we first started working together:

- Whole eggs are more nutritious than egg whites alone.
    - Both the fats and the cholesterol in the egg yolk have benefits and aren't the "bad guys" they have been called in the past.
    - Studies indicate that the consumption of 3 to 4 whole eggs per day is actually "heart healthy."
- Carbohydrates are neither good nor bad. Include them in your dietary intake based on necessity.

- You need carbohydrates/sugar to fuel your body, so if you have an active lifestyle, you need to consume them to perform optimally.

- Cooling down cooked foods that contain resistant starches is a great way to both minimize the available calories in those foods and feed the good bacteria in your gut.

- If you are performing high-intensity exercises, be sure you have sugar to burn, or you will learn the hard way like I did.

• A moderate to high amount of protein intake (30–40% of your total calories) helps with three key things while in a calorie deficit:

- Protein helps to spare muscle.

- Protein helps increase satiety— "makes you feel full."

- Protein has a relatively high TEF (Thermic Effect of Food)—"you will burn more calories breaking down protein than carbohydrates or fats."

• Coffee and other foods and drinks that contain caffeine can be used to reduce hunger, thereby reducing total food intake.

- - Caffeine's stimulant effect can also help mitigate the lethargy that sometimes comes with the reduced calorie intake used to achieve a fat loss goal.

- As best you can, try to eat mostly "whole foods" that have been alive as recently as possible. Basically, this helps to eliminate the highly processed foods that are way too calorie dense, lacking in essential vitamins and enzymes, and devoid of real nutritional value. You also get the benefit of a higher TEF as whole foods require more of the body's energy to break them down than processed foods do.

- Try to keep your macronutrients (carbohydrates, fats, and proteins) fairly balanced with a slight prioritization based on your specific lifestyle needs.

Percentage of calories by macronutrient

Type of person	Protein	Carbs	Fats
Average American	40%	30%	30%
Hungry	30%	30%	40%
Active	30%	40%	30%

- Regular people: If you have a fairly inactive lifestyle (read: the average American), your daily food should be composed of approximately 40% protein, 30% carbohydrates, and 30% fat. This balance provides enough carbohydrates and fats to fuel your life and proteins to keep your body from breaking down.

- Hungry people: If you find that you tend to be hungry all the time, shift these percentages around to prioritize more fats as they will help you feel fuller for longer, which would put you at 40% fat, 30% carbohydrates, and 30% protein.

- Active people: If your lifestyle is more active than the average person, your body needs and can use more carbohydrates, so your macronutrient balance should be closer to 40% carbohydrates, 30% protein, and 30% fat.

Section 3:

WHEN SHOULD YOU EAT TO MAXIMIZE RESULTS?

Knowing what to eat is only part of the equation for getting the weight loss results you are looking for. As it turns out, WHEN you eat can also make a huge difference in both how your body uses the foods that you consume and how it impacts the rest of your day.

So, how can you use purposeful timing of your meals to optimize feeling great, having lots of energy, AND still losing the excess body fat? As you might have guessed, it requires that you pay attention to YOUR life and implementing a few key concepts.

One of the major changes I had to make in my way of thinking when working with Jason was how frequently I ate. I, like most of you, have been in the habit of eating on a fairly consistent schedule:

- Breakfast in the morning before I headed to work.

- Lunch at work in the middle of the day.

- Dinner in the evening after I got home from work.

This typical three-meals-a-day schedule is how most Americans consume their food, and they don't ever really think twice about WHY they eat at these times, nor do they question if this is optimal for fueling their bodies or achieving their weight loss goals.

Science has shown us that neither the frequency of meals[33] nor the time of day[34] those meals are eaten has very much of an impact on your metabolism (the rate at which your body uses energy) or on losing fat.

Yes, I know, that is the OPPOSITE of what you have been told for years. It made my face crinkle up a little when I was first told that as well, but with

---

[33] Alhussain, M, M. A. Taylor and I. A. Macdonald. 2015. "Influence of the constancy of daily meal pattern on postprandial energy expenditure in healthy weight women"
[34] Almoosawi, S., et al. 2016. "Chrono-nutrition: a review of current evidence from observational studies on global trends in time-of-day of energy intake and its association with obesity"

more and more scientific research being done, we are learning that the old assumptions just don't ring true.

The differences in your metabolism and ability to lose fat based on whether you consume most of your calories in the morning or the evening are so tiny that they may as well be ignored, so you can focus on the far more important aspects of your food intake, like total calories and types of foods consumed.

Perhaps the most important thing to focus on when determining when you should be consuming your meals is your lifestyle.

Some people get cranky if they don't eat every few hours, so it may be best for them to eat more consistent, smaller meals just to maintain their mood. I have fairly hectic mornings myself getting my two children up and ready for school as well as getting myself ready to commute to work. This oftentimes makes it very tough to plan, prepare, and consume a meal that is in line with my goals, so I typically just grab a coffee on the way to the office.

Additionally, once I get to work I tend to get so involved in my projects that I can forget what time it is, and POOF it will already be half way through the day, and I have still had nothing to eat. I used to think this was terrible for me, but after sharing my experience with Jason, he reassured me that we could find a way to make my lifestyle work for me instead of against me.

This is where the concept of Intermittent Fasting came into play.

INTERMITTENT FASTING

You may have heard of this fairly new trend of intermittent fasting (IM) as it has become very popular over the last few years. There are dozens of books written about it and entire websites dedicated to its practice.

Essentially, the concept is that our bodies are made to go for relatively long periods of time (hours, days, and even weeks) with little to no food intake and still survive[35]. You have to remember, we as a species have only recently (the last 200 years or so) had readily available foods to the extent that we even had the option to overeat and accumulate excess body fat.

Throughout the vast majority of human evolution, we have had to adapt physiologically to the "hunter-gatherer" lifestyle, so we developed the ability to store food (as body fat) whenever we did

[35] Patterson, Ruth E., and Dorothy D. Sears. 2017. "Metabolic Effects of Intermittent Fasting"

manage to feast on some berries on a bush, fish in a stream, or any other bounty we came across.

Our bodies are made to switch between various sources of energy, two of which we have already discussed: carbohydrates/sugars and fats.

When they are readily available, these are the two preferred energy sources that your body will take advantage of, but in their absence (when fasting for an extended period of time), your body will convert stored fat into what are known as ketones and then release these into the bloodstream where they can be picked up by pretty much any cell and used as a form of energy[36]. Your body can survive for a pretty long time by using your stored body fat in this manner, making us a little more resilient than if we depended on sugar alone to fuel our bodies.

Speaking of ketones, in case you have been living under a rock for the last few years, the "ketogenic diet" trend that is currently all the rage encourages people to purposely put themselves into a state where they use these very ketones as fuel.

The keto diet proponents out there don't use starvation as the means to produce ketones, but rather they use a super-high-fat diet (75%+ of calories from fats!), which can kinda "trick" the

---

[36] Seimon, Radhika V., et al. 2015. "Do intermittent diets provide physiological benefits over continuous diets for weight loss? A systematic review of clinical trials"

body into thinking it's in a starvation state, thereby creating ketones from body fat[37].

This dietary trend is rather interesting in its claims and value propositions, but in general it is no more effective at helping someone to lose body fat than more moderate fat-/carbohydrate-intake diets that don't force your body into ketosis[38]. The keto diet does have some great benefits for people with Alzheimer's disease[39] or certain types of cancer[40], and even for people who suffer from certain types of seizures[41]. All of these are great reasons for looking into the keto diet, but they are not the focus of this book, so I'll just suggest you consult your physician if you are interested in learning more.

So, back to intermittent fasting.

When Jason introduced me to the concept of IM, he suggested it might be of value to me based on my

---

[37] Bueno, Nassib Bezerra, et al. 2013. "Very-low-carbohydrate ketogenic diet v. low-fat diet for long-term weight loss: a meta-analysis of randomised controlled trials"
[38] Gardner CD, et al. 2018. "Effect of Low-Fat vs. Low-Carbohydrate Diet on 12-Month Weight Loss in Overweight Adults and the Association with Genotype Pattern or Insulin Secretion: The DIETFITS Randomized Clinical Trial"
[39] Maciej Gasior, Michael A. Rogawski, and Adam L. Hartmana. 2006. "Neuroprotective and disease-modifying effects of the ketogenic diet"
[40] Bryan G. Allen, et al. 2014. "Ketogenic diets as an adjuvant cancer therapy: History and potential mechanism"
[41] Kristin W. Barañano, MD, PhD and Adam L. Hartman, MD. 2008. "The Ketogenic Diet: Uses in Epilepsy and Other Neurologic Illnesses"

specific lifestyle. What I learned was that, for my lifestyle, it was not only acceptable to go long periods of time without eating (remember, I usually only had a cup of coffee and wouldn't eat till late in the afternoon), but it was actually a good idea as it kept me from eating too many total calories.

The IM plan that ended up working best for me was to make every other weekday an IM day by going a full 24 hours without eating. It sounds extreme but hear me out.

As an example, I will eat normally on Sunday all day, and after I finish my Sunday evening dinner around 7 p.m., I will start my fast. This means I will go the eight hours of sleep with no food (no big deal, of course), and then I will only have black coffee in the morning on Monday and maybe another cup (or two!) of black coffee in the afternoon while I work. The caffeine in the coffee helps to keep my appetite at bay, and by the time I get home from work on Monday evening, it is about the 24-hour mark for my fast, so I will have dinner to break my "fast."

Seeing as how I typically enjoy eating foods that are higher in protein and fat for this first meal at the end of my fast—foods like steak, eggs, and avocados—I am TRULY, in every sense of the word, having "breakfast" for dinner!

Now, you understand why at the very beginning of this book I make the odd-sounding declaration "How I lost 45 lbs in 3 months eating a traditional American breakfast."

Not so odd-sounding now, is it?

In essence, using intermittent fasting as one of the many "tools" I factor into my day-to-day eating has helped me to NOT overeat, especially on the fasting days, thereby allowing me to maintain a fairly consistent calorie deficit and the amazing fat loss results that come with it.

For the purposes of this book, IM simply allows me to control when I eat and, of course, how much I eat. There really isn't any magic to it other than a planned-in-advance timeframe when I am not stuffing my face.

One additional thing to keep in mind with my particular situation and overall program is that I do high-intensity interval-training (HIIT) workouts a couple times a week, and that type of exercise requires my body to use sugar as its primary energy source. (The "30-Minute Overeasy System Exercise Program" we have included with this book is a form of this high-intensity interval training and is one of the fastest ways to make your body stronger, more conditioned, and in shape.)

To ensure I have the fuel my body needs to get me through these rigorous workouts, I strategically place my workouts on the days where I am NOT fasting to ensure I am fully fueled to have a great workout[42].

If I do a HIIT workout on the days that I fast, my blood sugar will probably be too low to sustain the activity, and I may end up becoming hypoglycemic (the fancy word for having low blood sugar) and getting light-headed. Not a good idea, so I simply plan my workouts according to my IM schedule, and all is good!

I learned this the hard way one day at Orangetheory during one of my fasts, when I nearly fainted 20 minutes into a high-intensity workout. I hadn't eaten anything for nearly 20 hours (since dinner the day before), so I was already low on blood sugar when I started my workout, and seeing how high-intensity exercise makes my body use primarily sugar as its fuel source, let's just say things didn't work out so well for me. Long story short: make sure to have some food/carbs before doing a high-intensity workout so you are properly fueled!

Sometimes, it's the simple things like this that make the most profound differences when trying to

---

[42] Hill, James O., et al. 1989. "Evaluation of an alternating-calorie diet with and without exercise in the treatment of obesity"

achieve your fat loss goals. I hope this recurring theme is something you are picking up on: fat loss really can be "simple" or "easy" if you just understand the basic concepts and apply them to your specific lifestyle as opposed to trying to force your lifestyle to conform to a rigid "diet" that bastardizes one or more types of food.

SATIETY

As I have talked about previously, whenever you consume proteins or fats, your body releases the hormone CCK (cholecystokinin), which makes you feel full[43], and this is, of course, a nugget of information that can be used strategically to your advantage if you stop and think about it for a moment.

If you are one of those people who works a typical 9-5 job, and you find that a few hours after lunch you are already starving again, it would be a great idea to switch up how much protein and/or fat you are packing into your lunch meal or your snacks[44]. Simply adding a whole hard-boiled egg to your lunch or grabbing some almonds for a snack can

---

[43] Näslund, Erik, and Per M. Hellström. 2007. Appetite signaling: from gut peptides and enteric nerves to brain"
[44] Bowen, et al. 2006. Appetite regulatory hormone responses to various dietary proteins differ by body mass index status despite similar reductions in ad libitum energy intake"

help to stimulate the release of CCK in your body, which will keep you from getting overly hungry, which in turn leads to most people overeating once they are finally off work.

As it turns out, the majority of people tend to overeat in the evenings after they pushed through a long day of school, work, or household responsibilities. This is probably why it is so common to hear silly things like "Don't eat after 6 p.m. because it causes weight gain". The reality here is that it really doesn't matter when you eat, as long as you are NOT overeating[45]. This becomes all too challenging for a lot of Americans when they find themselves extremely hungry, in part due to consuming predominantly carbohydrates throughout the day, as we know carbohydrates don't help much in the way of satiety.

If you are overly hungry, there is a HIGH likelihood that you'll overeat, and that just is not conducive to your weight loss goals.

Swapping in some healthy fats and proteins earlier in the day, at lunch time, or as a snack can really help to prevent overeating at dinner time, and therefore you will be well on your way to losing those extra pounds that you have been trying to get

---

[45] Davoodi, Sayed Hossein, et al. 2014. "Calorie Shifting Diet Versus Calorie Restriction Diet: A Comparative Clinical Trial Study"

rid of for far too long. Couple this with a little less "boredom" eating while you sit in front of the TV late at night, and you'll have a one-two punch at the heart of what has probably caused you to gain the weight in the first place: too much food that you really didn't need to consume.

I don't want to neglect some of the great carbohydrate sources out there as being unhelpful in the fight against weight loss, hypertension, and diabetes, as the truth is that all types of vegetables can be a great tool in your weight loss journey.

In all honesty, filling yourself up on vegetables and other high-volume, high-nutrient (vitamins, minerals, polyphenols, etc.), low-energy (calories) foods is one of the fundamental principles of weight management[46]. Plant matter like vegetables, fruit, legumes (beans), and tubers (potatoes) all contain a lot of fiber, both soluble and insoluble. Eating a big old salad can be just as effective in reducing hunger as the CCK released when consuming fats and proteins, as the bulk of the fiber actually helps to stretch out the stomach, which in turn signals the body to feel full. Even if you have terrible eating habits to begin with, simply adding in a big salad or a couple servings of vegetables to your daily food

---

[46] Woods, Stephen C. 2004. "Gastrointestinal satiety signals I. An overview of gastrointestinal signals that influence food intake"

intake will make you feel fuller, which means you will eat less of the bad stuff and start losing weight.

One other super-simple way you can control your hunger to ensure you don't overeat is to slow down the actual eating process. While the hormone CCK is great for aiding in satiety when you consume foods with proteins and fats in them, there are other factors at play in the actual mechanics of food consumption that can help you. Chewing your food up more slowly signals the brain to feel fuller sooner[47], and that can be another simple tool available to you when looking to shed those extra pounds.

CARBOHYDRATES FOR FUEL

Choosing a specific time to eat more fats and proteins so that you can control your hunger is a great tool you can use to your advantage, but what if you happen to have a really active lifestyle and need to keep yourself fueled for optimal performance?

As you recall, carbohydrate, more specifically sugar (glucose), is the primary fuel source for most of your body's systems, so if you are looking to

---

[47] Campbell, Caroline L., Ty B. Wagoner, and E. Allen Foegeding. 2016. "Designing foods for satiety: The roles of food structure and oral processing in satiation and satiety"

improve your performance during physical activities (exercising, labor-intensive job), it is a good idea to purposely consume some carbohydrates prior to those activities[48].

Let's say you work in manual labor, and you feel like you are just dragging through the day due to low energy. This would be a good example for when you should purposely eat some complex carbohydrates (starchy foods like potatoes, rice, grains, and beans) a few hours prior to the activity.

The reason for eating these foods a couple hours before the activity is that it takes time to digest the starches and turn them into sugar before it is absorbed and available to be distributed via the bloodstream. Complex carbohydrates/starches help to maintain elevated blood levels of sugars for hours after they are eaten, and this means fuel for your labor-intensive job so you don't get all worn out[49].

If you are looking to boost the effort you can put forth in your workout, or if you just don't have the time to eat hours before an activity, you can just consume some simple sugars like a piece of fruit or some juice, and it will digest and absorb much

---

[48] Paolo C Colombani, et al. 2013. "Carbohydrates and exercise performance in non-fasted athletes: A systematic review of studies mimicking real-life"
[49] JA Hawley, et al. 1997. "Carbohydrate-Loading and Exercise Performance"

faster than starches, therefore making it available for use within minutes as opposed to hours[50].

I like to eat a couple clementines before I head out for a HIIT workout, as I usually haven't consumed any carbs earlier that day, and this boy isn't gonna have another faint spell.

The claim that sugar is "bad for you," or that it causes weight gain just by existing, is just outright nonsense. Purposefully choosing when and how much sugar to consume can be an incredibly useful skill that allows you to get the most out of your day-to-day lifestyle, and it can even contribute to your weight loss goals. Just as is the case with all of the other macronutrients, picking and choosing the best sources of carbohydrates, as well as WHEN and HOW MUCH to consume, makes all the difference between "bad" and "good."

COFFEE AS AN APPETITE SUPPRESSANT

Something we have already talked about before, coffee, can play a potent role in the timing of your food intake.

---

[50] Wong JM, Jenkins DJ. 2007. "Carbohydrate digestibility and metabolic effects"

As we have discussed before, the caffeine in coffee is a central nervous system stimulant (makes you alert and feel full of energy), and one of the "side effects" of that stimulant effect is that it tends to be an appetite suppressant for most people[51].

This is why a lot of people who drink coffee first thing in the morning tend to NOT eat breakfast or to eat a smaller portion as they just aren't that hungry, thanks to the coffee. This is neither good nor bad, but if you understand the effects that the caffeine in coffee and other beverages can have on you, it empowers you to be able to use them as a purposeful tool.

If you find you get hungry at certain times of day, having a caffeinated beverage can help to calm that hunger and keep you on track with your food intake, especially if you are on a calorie-restricted dietary intake with a fat loss goal.

IN SUMMARY

So, what are the key takeaways when it comes to timing your food intake for maximum fat loss and optimal performance throughout your day?

---

[51] Tamara Bakuradze, et al. 2014. "Four-week coffee consumption affects energy intake, satiety regulation, body fat, and protects DNA integrity"

Let's break them down here:

- The standard three-meals-per-day (breakfast, lunch, and dinner) timing of food intake may not be optimal for a lot of people and can in fact contribute to gaining weight if you have a sedentary lifestyle.

    a. Frequent small meals are no more valuable than one large meal per day for a fat loss goal.

- Intermittent fasting is one method of controlling when you consume food by limiting your food intake to certain times of day.

    a. Fasting forces your body to use fat as fuel by converting it into ketone that your cells can use to fuel their activity.

    b. If you choose to use IM, make sure to plan your exercise/physical activity around the times when you are eating.

- Strategically choosing foods throughout the day can help keep you satiated so you won't get cranky or overeat. Either/both of the options below might work for you:

    a. Eat foods higher in healthy fats and protein as they release CCK to aid in early meal termination.

    b. Eat leafy greens and other fibrous vegetables as the bulk of the fiber helps to stretch out the stomach, which in turn signals the body to feel full.

- Time the consumption of carbohydrates to fuel your activities such as manual labor or a workout.

    a. Consume complex carbohydrates a couple hours prior to activity to allow for full digestion and absorption.

    b. Consume simple sugars 30 to 60 minutes prior to activity as they digest and absorb very quickly.

- Drinking coffee or some other caffeinated beverage can help to suppress your appetite, thereby preventing you from overeating.

Section 4:

HOW MUCH FOOD SHOULD YOU BE CONSUMING TO ACHIEVE YOUR GOALS?

In case you haven't been paying attention so far, there is a recurring theme in what we have covered.

First, we talked about WHAT to eat, and then we moved on to WHEN you should be eating it. Now, we are going to cover the third pillar for nutrition success: HOW MUCH you should be eating.

Quite honestly, this is actually the most important factor when it comes to losing fat, gaining muscle, or otherwise improving your health. Total calories consumed as compared to the total number of calories used in a given day is the basic equation that everyone must solve if they truly want to achieve their weight loss goal, as no matter the quality of your foods, or when you consume them, the laws of physics always have their way with you.

In this case, we are talking about the first law of thermodynamics: Energy can neither be created nor destroyed; it can only change forms. What this means in practical terms is that as you continue to add energy (food) to your body (calories-in), if there isn't an equal amount of energy leaving your body, burned through activity (calories-out), you will grow larger.

Sadly, that growth doesn't tend to be rippling muscle; rather, it comes in the form of unwanted extra body fat. Bummer!

If you want to lose fat, the basic equation we need to adhere to is making sure that you burn more calories every day than you consume, in essence creating an energy deficit.

Where does the extra energy that you use in a given day come from, if not your food?

Reach down and poke that squishy stuff on your belly to best answer this question. We store the extra food we eat that we didn't use in the form of body fat. Our amazing bodies are simply saving the extra food/energy we consumed for a "rainy day" in case we need it. In order to lose your unwanted extra body fat, you simply need to create that "rainy day" situation via one or both of the following actions:

- Eat less (calories-in)

- Move more (calories-out)

The optimal way to go about getting rid of those unwanted pounds it is to incorporate both of these actions, but the truth is that the vast majority of fat loss comes from controlling your food intake[52].

Exercise and overall increased activity have a multitude of great benefits, but that is the topic of a totally different book. For the purposes of this book, we will focus on the calorie-in part of the equation.

CALORIES-IN

So, all you have to do is eat less total calories than you use every day, and you'll lose body fat like it's going out of style?

Yes, it is really that simple, but simple doesn't necessarily mean easy. If it were easy, everyone

---

[52] KE Foster-Schubert, CM Alfano, CR Duggan, L Xiao, KL Campbell, A Kong, C Bain, CY Wang, G Blackburn, and A McTiernan. 2012. "Effect of diet and exercise, alone or combined, on weight and body composition in overweight-to-obese post-menopausal women"

would be doing it, and there wouldn't be an epidemic of obesity in the United States. Obviously, it will require effort on your part, but you already knew that, so I'm not telling you anything new. In essence, the goal of this book is to simplify all of the noise out there in the nutrition world that might steer you off course, preventing you from getting the results you deserve. I will be the first to tell you people can overcomplicate tracking their calories-in and turn it into a complete mess.

There are basically three ways most people keep track of their calories-in:

1. Guesstimate using familiar objects to gauge approximate calories—this is the least accurate method but the easiest to stick with.

2. Weigh/measure the foods that you eat regularly and try to stick to eating those same foods over and over— works well for people who don't mind the monotony.

3. Weigh/measure everything, all the time— this is the most effective for those who are serious about results, but it can become a little tedious.

Which one will work best for you? That really depends on your personality type and your lifestyle.

If you are the type who enjoys controlling all the variables in your life, weighing and measuring everything you eat every single day may be the best way to go. This method will give you very accurate measurements and can lead to great results if you are able to stick with it.

People who have very regimented, highly scheduled lives tend to eat the same things over and over to begin with, so it makes sense for them to weigh and measure those foods one time and simply eat them repetitively. You will find that a lot of physique athletes, like bodybuilders, tend towards this type of regimen. They will determine the exact foods and amounts they need and prepare an entire week's worth of those specific foods in advance and eat the same thing every day.

I personally prefer a little more variety in my life when it comes to eating, and I also don't want to have to weigh and measure everything I consume, so I operate best with the first option: guesstimating using familiar objects to gauge their approximate calories. Jason shared a very unique technique with me that he learned from one of the foremost authorities on nutrition, precisionnutrition.com[53]. This seems to be the best way for the majority of people out there who are trying to lose some body fat as it doesn't require

---

[53] Precision Nutrition Calorie Counting Guide - https://www.precisionnutrition.com/calorie-control-guide

any special measuring devices. The preferred familiar object to use for this process is something you always have with you no matter where you are: your hand!

In order to determine your portion sizes for each meal, all you have to do is remember the following "measurements":

- A veggie portion the size of your fist.
- A carbohydrate portion that fills your hand.
- A protein portion the size of your palm.
- A fat portion the size of your thumb.

The great thing about using your own hand to do this type of guesstimating is that your hand is personalized to YOUR body. Larger people have larger hands, and smaller people have smaller hands, so the portions are already "customized" to you.

Yes, I know, some people have hands that aren't directly proportional to their body size, but keep in mind this is guesstimating, so we aren't pretending this is an exact science. Most people don't measure their food at all, so this method is a HUGE improvement.

Assuming that you eat three times a day (you can obviously adjust that number to fit your lifestyle), your daily intake will look like the following based on gender:

For men:

- 2 veggie portions the size of your fist.
- 2 carbohydrate portions that fills your hand.
- 2 protein portions the size of your palm.
- 2 fat portions the size of your thumb.

For women:

- 1 veggie portion the size of your fist.
- 1 carbohydrate portion that fills your hand.
- 1 protein portion the size of your palm.
- 1 fat portion the size of your thumb.

Keep in mind that the amounts of carbohydrate and fat based foods should be adjusted based on how active you are (more carbohydrates if you're more active, less if you aren't), and how much hunger you are experiencing (more fat if you feel hungry all the time, less if you don't).

Protein food sources are things like eggs, fish, beef, chicken, pork, dairy products, and beans. Vegetables are items like salad greens, broccoli, cauliflower, and asparagus. Carbohydrate food sources are items like fruits, grains, pasta, and potatoes. Finally, fat food sources are things like seeds, nuts, and oils.

BALANCED NUTRITION

These portions are designed to provide an approximate macronutrient profile of 40% protein, 30% carbohydrates, and 30% fats that works out great for the average person looking to lose body fat. This ratio is NOT fixed in stone, but it is meant to give a far more balanced mixture of nutrition to your body than you probably have had up to this point[54].

Some simple adjustments to the above guidelines allow you to customize your macronutrient profile to one that is best suited for your lifestyle as outlined here:

1. Regular people: If you have a fairly inactive lifestyle (the average American), your daily food should be composed of approximately 40% protein, 30% carbohydrates, and 30% fat. This balance provides enough carbohydrates and fats to fuel your life and enough proteins to keep your body from breaking down. This is what the standard recommendation of portions is based on.

2. Hungry people: If you find that you tend to be hungry all of the time, shift these

---

[54] Fulgoni VL 3rd. 2008. "Current protein intake in America: analysis of the National Health and Nutrition Examination Survey, 2003-2004"

percentages around to prioritize more fats as they will help you to feel fuller for longer, which would put you at 40% fat, 30% carbohydrates, and 30% protein. To adjust to this ratio, simply drop off a couple of the carb servings and make sure to have all of your fat servings.

3. Active people: If your lifestyle is more active than the average person, you body needs and can use more carbohydrates, so your macronutrient balance should be closer to 40% carbohydrates, 30% protein, and 30% fat. To adjust to this ratio, simply drop off one of the fat servings and make sure to have all of your carbohydrate servings.

The standard American diet (SAD) typically consists of about 70% carbs, 15% protein, and 15% fat, so by decreasing the excessive amount of carbs and increasing the other macronutrients, we are helping to decrease hunger, minimize binge-eating, and maximize the raw materials needed for your body to operate optimally[55]. There is no perfect ratio of these macronutrients, but the goal here isn't perfection but rather progress towards your fat loss goals.

---

[55] Bowen, et al. 2006. "Appetite regulatory hormone responses to various dietary proteins differ by body mass index status despite similar reductions in ad libitum energy intake"

Ultimately, this is a great starting point for someone looking to change their lifestyle habits with food consumption as it is easy to remember and requires no special tools. No, it is NOT the most accurate method of measuring your food, but that isn't what we are going for at this point.

Transitioning from NOT measuring your food at all to now paying close enough attention to purposefully allocate portions of individual food types using your hand is a HUGE shift in the right direction. A recurring theme I have been trying to share with you is that in order for any of these simple nutrition concepts to work for you, they must be flexible enough to fit into YOUR lifestyle. This is where most diet plans go wrong—they try to force you to fit into their "box" as opposed to having the flexibility that allows for your unique lifestyle with all of its specific demands.

If you don't like to work out and have a sedentary lifestyle overall, just cut out one or two of the cupped hands of carbohydrate-dense foods as you really don't need them. If you are someone who is always hungry no matter what you eat, make sure to include the recommended "thumb" of fat-dense foods at every meal to help keep you satiated. It's really that easy to customize your food intake for your unique lifestyle, and that is a major reason why I have gotten such incredible results, and so have the thousands of people who eat in this manner.

Once you have become proficient with the "hand" method, it would be wise to progress to measuring your foods a little more accurately.

Why, you ask?

Well, at first, ANY change in dietary intake, such as using the hand method, will bring about results. You will start to see and feel changes in your body within the first week or two, and that is great!

The problem is that once your body adapts to these nutritional adjustments, the inaccuracy of the wiggle room that is inherent to the hand method will start to become more apparent, and your results will begin to slow down. In order to continue to see the amazing fat loss results you want, you're going to have to "tighten" things up, and that means progressing to the next phase of measurement. How you go about this is your choice, again based on lifestyle. Upgrading from the hand method to one of the other methods is the next step in really gaining control over your food so that you can get maximum results and ensure lifelong maintenance.

Remember, this is NOT a "quick fix" or a band aid on the situation but rather a lifestyle adjustment meant to get you the fat loss you desire and KEEP the fat off. That means developing new habits and ways of looking at your food. Whether you choose to meal-prep and only measure your foods once a week or to weigh and measure everything, the goal isn't to do as such forever, but rather only do it for as long as it takes for you to establish new habits that help you to have an improved relationship with what foods you eat, when you eat them, and how much of them you consume. The best way to do this is to track them.

KEEPING RECORDS

Some people like to use a journal to track their food intake, others prefer using an app on their computer or phone. Whatever method you choose to fit your lifestyle, the benefit remains the same: by tracking everything, you are not only able to see what is working and what isn't working, you are also all but guaranteeing your own results.

I personally can't guarantee your results with The Overeasy System because I can't guarantee that you'll actually do any of the things recommended here. If I could twist your arm and force you to follow the plan, then I could guarantee results, but that's just not realistic.

The best plan in the world is of no value if it isn't followed. By measuring your food and tracking it, you are essentially holding yourself accountable to doing the things you know are best for your fat loss goals and overall health.

ACCOUNTABILITY

Accountability is an incredibly powerful tool in achieving success. When I first met Jason at the gym, and we had our very first personal training session, he sat me down and told me what he believed his value as a fitness professional was in helping me to get the success I so desired:

- Education - Learn the things needed to change my lifestyle/behaviors to get results.

- Motivation - Maintain focus on the end goal and celebrate the little "wins" along the way.

- Accountability - Keep track of what's working and what's not working, so I can make adjustments when needed.

The goal of this book is to help educate you so that you have the information needed to actually change your relationship with food and modify how you eat so you can achieve the goals you have set forth.

Part of that education is letting you know that in order to lose all the body fat you want based on your unique goals, you are going to have to hold yourself accountable to actually follow through with the things you've learned here.

There are two basic forms of accountability:

1. Intrinsic accountability - This is YOU holding yourself accountable by tracking what you do each day to move towards your goals. This requires a LOT of discipline.

2. Extrinsic accountability - This is other people helping to keep you on course during your journey towards your goals. This doesn't require nearly as much discipline, as you have other people to help you.

I personally am really disciplined and am able to keep myself accountable by tracking all my food, but I CHOOSE to add in some extrinsic accountability as it is very motivating having other people "along for the ride."

I do this in a few different ways. One thing I have found works great for me is tracking my food in a nutrition app on my phone that has a built-in community of other people working towards their health and fitness goals. This is a great combination of intrinsic and extrinsic accountability as I have to be responsible for measuring my foods and entering them every day, but I also have the benefit of interacting with a bunch of other people who are doing the same thing, and that keeps me on point, lest they find out I've been slacking and give me a hard time (in good fun, of course).

Using an app to track my food and to interact with a community of other people on a similar journey has helped to keep me engaged in this process and even given me something to look forward to.

I really enjoy when I do my weekly weigh-ins to see my progress as I can share it with my friends in the app, and they always cheer me on, which, of course, is super motivating. I am a software engineer by trade, so once I found out how much I enjoyed using an app to track my food, I decided I would put together my own app that included an entire community of users like myself because I wanted to customize it for all the things I felt would really help me and everyone else to be successful.

The other thing I found works wonders for keeping me focused on achieving my goals with my nutrition was joining a Facebook group. I do a lot of work on the computer and use Facebook regularly to connect with like-minded people.

Finally, I share my lifestyle journey on social media. I find that by continuously putting myself out there, it may be motivating others who are on a similar journey, and I don't want to let them down.

IN SUMMARY

We covered a lot of information when discussing how much food you should be consuming to maximize fat loss and optimize performance throughout your day.

Let's review it here:

- Calories-in versus calories-out is the MOST important factor in achieving your fat loss goals. You can create a calorie deficit by doing one or both of the following:

    - Eat less (calories-in)

    - Move more (calories-out)

- There are three basic ways to track your calories-in:

    - Guesstimate using your hand to gauge approximate calories—this is the least accurate method but the easiest to stick with.

    - Weigh/measure the foods that you eat regularly and try to stick to eating those same foods over and over—works well for people who don't mind the monotony.

- Weigh/measure everything, all the time—this is the most effective method for those who are serious about results, but it can become a little tedious.
- Starting with the "hand method" is a great way to transition from not measuring your food at all. All you have to remember is the following:
    - Your palm determines your protein portions.
    - Your fist determines your vegetable portions.
    - Your cupped hand determines your carb portions.
    - Your thumb determines your fat portions.
- Assuming you will eat four times per day, follow these guidelines for the "hand method":
    - For men:
        i. 2 palms of protein-dense foods with each meal
        ii. 2 fists of vegetables with each meal

- iii. 2 cupped hands of carb-dense foods with *most* meals
- iv. 2 entire thumbs of fat-dense foods with *most* meals

○ For women:

- i. 1 palm of protein-dense foods with each meal
- ii. 1 fist of vegetables with each meal
- iii. 1 cupped hand of carb-dense foods with *most* meals
- iv. 1 entire thumb of fat-dense foods with *most* meals

• Adjust your macronutrient profile to fit your specific lifestyle, similar to the following:

Type of person	Protein	Carbs	Fats
Average American	40%	30%	30%
Hungry	30%	30%	40%
Active	30%	40%	30%

- Track your food intake to ensure you are getting optimal results and to hold yourself accountable. Accountability comes in two forms:
    - Intrinsic accountability
    - Extrinsic accountability
- Use a combination of intrinsic and extrinsic accountability to maximize your opportunity for success by doing the following:
    - Track your foods using a nutrition app and engage the community to help hold you accountable and motivate you with your successes.
    - Join and engage with The Overeasy System Facebook group to learn what is working for the other group members, find new recipe ideas, and keep up with the latest nutrition information.
    - Share your journey via social media.

Section 5:

THE OVEREASY SYSTEM

Throughout my fat loss journey, the biggest changes have been with my mindset and the way I view food.

Like many Americans, I viewed food like this: "LIVE TO EAT!"

However, how we should view food, and how I view it now, is like this:

EAT TO LIVE

Eating for survival is the main way we should view food: We consume food to stay alive.

Through intermittent fasting, I've learned that you'll be 100% fine if you don't eat for an extended period of time. So, the amount of food we need to survive is a lot less than most people consume on a daily basis. Just because breakfast, lunch, and dinner are the norm doesn't mean we have to follow it. Following it is how we got into this obesity epidemic anyways, isn't it?

EAT FOR PURPOSE

The second step is understanding how and why you should eat food for optimal performance.

If you are going to exercise, you need a certain amount of energy to have an optimal workout. If you perform manual labor, you'll need to consume more than someone who sits at a desk all day. Building muscle? You probably need more protein. Going to do a HIIT workout? Make sure you have sugar to burn. Gonna binge-watch TV all day? Stop eating like a jerk.

Start off by understanding why you are eating in the first place.

LIVE TO EAT

Finally, eat for the love of food! You have to be able to eat the foods you love if you expect to have a healthy lifestyle that will last forever. I've been able to enjoy the foods I love by following the first two mindsets above and still drop 45 lbs while doing so. And I did this through the football and holiday season, when most Americans are packing on the pounds.

> **Eat to Live >> Eat for Purpose >> Live to Eat**

If you are able to unlock this mindset, it is the key to a successful and healthy lifestyle.

Now that we understand the key principles of nutrition, I have put together a simple guide you can follow to live The Overeasy Life.

1. Learn what your basal metabolic rate (BMR) is. This is the rate at which your body uses energy while at rest to keep vital functions going, such as breathing and keeping warm. Basically, BMR is the amount of calories you burn on a daily basis if you did zero activity.

    a. You can calculate your BMR by using the calculator at http://www.bmi-calculator.net/bmr-calculator/ or simply googling BMR calculator.

    b. Now, take a look at your favorite foods and see how much of them you can consume within your BMR. For instance, I love chicken wings, and a wing at BW3 is about 72 calories. So, if all I ate were those wings in a day, I could eat 28 wings based on my BMR (and nothing else). Practice this exercise with all types of foods and you'll begin to get a grasp of how much you can actually eat without going into calorie excess.

2. Start eating **breakfast for dinner** a few times per week to help increase the amount of protein (steak and eggs) you are getting and add some more fat to your diet (eggs, avocados, nuts). The additional protein will help keep your total calorie intake down (remember: thermal effect of food), which along with the additional fat will help you feel more full, eliminating those late-night cravings so that you eat less overall.

3. Fast three times per week from dinner to dinner. After two to three weeks, you will teach the brain that you don't need to eat breakfast, lunch, and dinner like we have been doing all our lives. Moving forward, you'll be able to decide when is a good time to skip an unnecessary meal.

4. Start eating more whole foods in the form of fruits, vegetables, and protein sources like chicken, fish, or beef. Opt for an apple instead of apple juice. Did you know that it takes three whole apples to make a cup of apple juice? Now, think about how full you

would get after eating three apples compared to chugging down a glass of apple juice. The fiber in the whole apples would fill your stomach and make you feel fuller, plus there is a MUCH higher thermic effect of food with eating whole apples compared to apple juice[56]. Is it starting to sink in? Ever hear of someone getting fat eating fruits and vegetables? Yeah... me neither.

5. Eat carbs for a purpose. If you live an active lifestyle, then add more carbs to your diet. If you sit on your ass and don't work out, limit the carbs you eat and eat more fats and protein. And remember, DO NOT work out while fasting. Please, break your fast with some carbohydrates if you are going to exercise. I don't need you fainting at the gym like I did.

That's it. The system is meant to be easy to follow. I've tried to simplify what we have over complicated throughout the years. That's where the name Overeasy comes from... well, that and because I love to eat my eggs that way.

---

[56] Barr SB, Wright JC. 2010. "Postprandial energy expenditure in whole-food and processed-food meals: implications for daily energy expenditure"

Section 6:

THE LOWDOWN AND DIRTY TRICKS YOU CAN FOLLOW

I've adapted these simple techniques into my everyday lifestyle, and they have really helped me to control my calorie intake and get amazing fat loss results. Check them all out and see which ones might fit into your lifestyle and help you to do the same.

Fast During the Work Week

My fasting schedule has me not eating anything from dinner to dinner on Monday, Wednesday, and Friday during the work week. Seeing how busy most of us are during the week with school, work, and family, I've found that it's a lot easier to go extended periods of time without eating when I am already busy as my mind is preoccupied. Having this schedule also helps to get me "back on track" on Mondays after a tough weekend as I am less likely to cheat on one of my fasting days during the week than I would on a weekend.

Fast Before a Calorie Bomb

I fast when I'm going to be drinking, going to go out for dinner, going to a party, or attending an event, even if it lands on a day other than Monday, Wednesday, or Friday.

That's right, I could end up fasting for four, five, or maybe even six days in a week, depending on my social life. But, why consume breakfast or lunch when you know you're going to eat like an asshole and drink like a fish? In the past, I would eat regularly, then have these calorie explosions on top of it, which would slowly increase my weight over the years.

By cutting out the unnecessary meals before I participated in these calorie-laden activities, I instantly cut out tons of calories throughout the year that I would have normally consumed, thereby allowing me to continue tailgating at Dolphins football games, going on a brew bus with my friends, or even eating at one of my favorite restaurants with a Tito's and Soda in hand, of course. Real life means sometimes being able to "indulge," and instead of pretending like you won't ever do that again, simply plan ahead and cut some calories out to make up the difference.

Switch to Vodka Soda

I have switched my alcoholic beverage of choice to vodka soda with lime. I love craft beer, especially a nice hoppy IPA, but the calories in these types of beers can be nearly double the calories in vodka, plus soda water has no calories.

With lighter beers, the calories are comparable to a vodka soda, but you tend to drink twice as many to get to your "happy place," which means you are consuming double the amount of calories anyways.

So, by making the switch, I'm drinking a lower-calorie beverage, with a higher concentration of alcohol, which has allowed me to enjoy my cocktails on a regular basis and still get the fat loss results I wanted.

Remember when I told you about my 30-day experiment with not drinking any alcohol? It didn't work, but this sure did.

Eating That High-Fat Breakfast for Dinner

Like I mentioned, my go-to meal when breaking a fast is a nice high-fat breakfast at dinner.

I either go for steak and eggs with avocados, or eggs, bacon, and avocados. I stay away from carbohydrates with either option. These high-fat breakfast meals keep me feeling full off a single meal that day and helps me stay away from consuming anything later at night.

Keep Fruits and Vegetables at Home for Snacks

When I'm feeling hungry and have to snack on something, I stick to whole foods in the form of fruits and vegetables. I keep an abundance of fruits like clementines, apples, bananas, strawberries, and grapes at the house for this reason. I also make sure I have a large pack of carrots in the fridge, as I like to snack on those when I'm really hungry—they are a bit more dense than the fruit options but super-low in calories.

Remember, whole foods like these take more energy to break down than processed foods like chips, cereal, candy, and even juice. You must refrain from those foods in times of hunger and opt for whole foods instead.

Fast on the Road

When I travel, especially for work, I tend to fast during the day, as I'm usually busy with meetings, lectures, or working on something, so all I need is a bunch of coffee to get me through the day.

From years of experience, I know that I'll be attending dinners and cocktail hours during the evenings, so there is no reason for me to consume additional calories at breakfast or lunch. I also know darn well there's 0% chance that I work out while traveling.

I follow this routine regularly while on the road, especially when attending a conference.

For the Love, Not for Boredom

If you're eating for the love of eating, and you have calories to spare, go ahead and indulge, but make sure you're eating it for the right reason, not because you're bored.

Section 7:

INFLUENTIAL THOUGHTS FROM INFLUENTIAL PEOPLE

As I have said before, I like to incorporate "extrinsic accountability" by sharing my fat loss journey on social media. I talk about my own challenges and the things that are working for me, and I get a lot of feedback on what works for other people too. Along the way, I have made "cyber-friends" with a whole slew of health- and fitness-minded social influencers (basically, people who have either achieved great fitness success themselves or who help others to get results), and I have asked them to share with me their best advice for someone looking to lose fat and change their life. Here are some of the best pieces of advice I received.

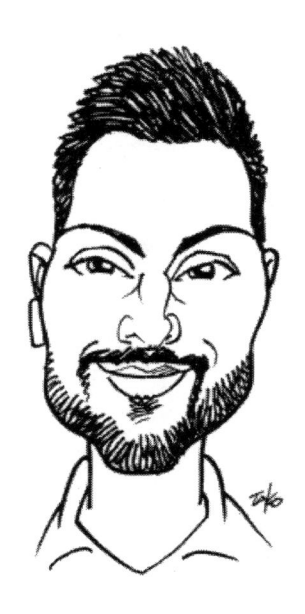

Carter Good
(IG: @cartergood)

His advice is to remember that, regardless of how long it takes you to lose weight, you'll spend most of your life maintaining it. So, don't focus too much on speed. Rather, focus on building a plan you can see yourself enjoying in the long run.

My Favorite Quote

"Don't be the Rabbit... Embrace the Turtle!"

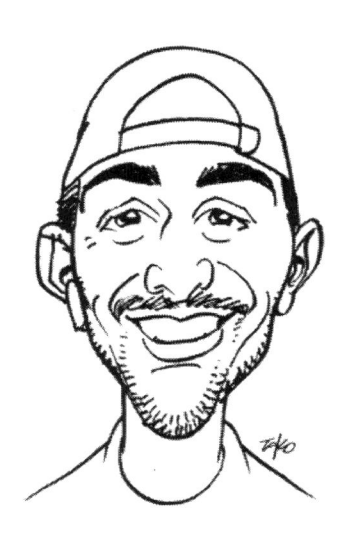

Jordan Syatt

(IG: @syattfitness)

Jordan had this to share. The not-so-marketable truth about fat loss is it's not easy. It's not quick. It's not fun or glamorous or noble.

Fat loss sucks. Straight up, it sucks. There are ways to make it less suck-y and more sustainable. You don't need to eliminate everything in your life, and you're absolutely able to lose fat without starving yourself. And you can 100% lose fat while having fun and living life.

But, the mental side of fat loss is what most people

overlook. It never goes as quickly as you want. You regularly feel like you're messing up. You often doubt yourself and your ability to stay on track. You sometimes feel like you're missing out on social events and struggle to find the balance between being strict enough to achieve your goals and being flexible enough to enjoy life.

The good news is all these struggles are normal. We all go through them. And with enough time, effort, dedication, and patience, you can and will come out on the other side, fully understanding how to stay lean year-round without ever having these feelings again.

But there's a difference. A difference between those who succeed and those who don't. And the difference lies solely in your ability to fail… and get up and try again.

Because you will go off track. You will make mistakes. You will have days and weeks and months that don't go your way. And that's OK. You will come out on top. You will win. You will succeed. I promise. Just as long as you're willing to keep getting back up and trying again and again and again. Because the only way to guarantee failure is to quit.

So, don't quit. Grit your teeth. Stand back up. And keep on fighting. You got this.

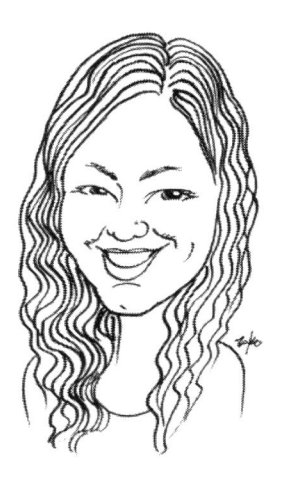

Lexi Reed

(@fatgirlfedup)

Lexi is truly an inspiration. She has lost over 300 lbs. during her fat loss journey. She shared with me the key to success was to not focus on how far you have to go but focus on each day. To start small and small changes will add up to big results!

My Favorite Quote

"Never Miss a Monday!"

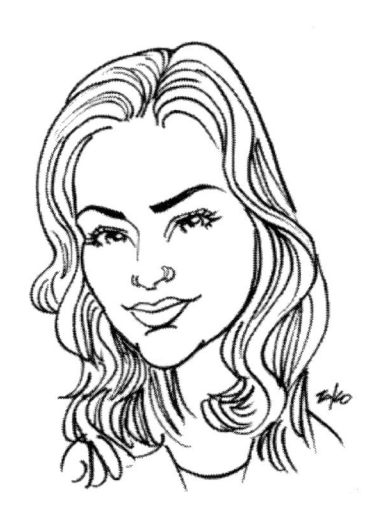

Sarah Nicole

(@thebirdspapaya)

Sarah's biggest piece of advice is to let go of the scale numbers and the sizes involved. Truly allow your health to be first and the weight loss a side effect of that healthy lifestyle. Your body knows where it should land, and in getting to know your body through a renewed relationship with it and with food, you'll discover what suits you best. Don't seek constant motivation but rely on your drive and your choice. Every day, let it be a decision that you own and are proud of.

Ultimately, don't let this be a lifestyle stemming from self-hate but rather a beautiful relationship with yourself stemming from self-love. Then, the destination won't matter so much—your happiness and health will.

> **My Favorite Quote**
>
> "Confidence isn't walking into a room thinking you're better than everyone else. It's walking in and not having to compare yourself to anyone at all."

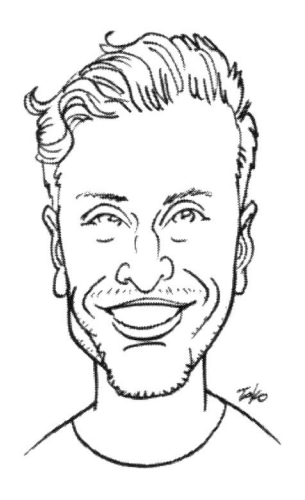

Matt Fox

(@mattycfox)

Matt is a cancer survivor, and for him, it all comes down to the fact that you need a goal, and you need to break those goals down into smaller goals (stepping stones) so you have a clear path. Don't overcomplicate things, just stay consistent—goals help you do that.

> **My Favorite Quote**
>
> "You gotta celebrate the little wins in life whenever they come along. It's too easy to dwell on negative things or stress on issues that don't matter, that we forget to be grateful for the amazing things we have."

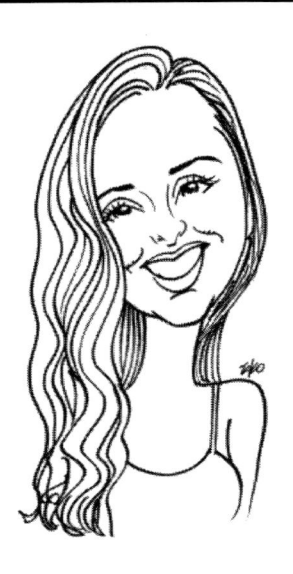

Mallory King

(@mallorykingfitness)

The advice she gives is to make a promise to yourself that you'll never give up. No matter how many times you fall down or mess up or feel like you'll never get there, the only thing that will ensure you don't make it to your goal is giving up. Keep going!

My Favorite Quote

"There's a recipe to successfully reaching a goal: positivity, persistence, and patience."

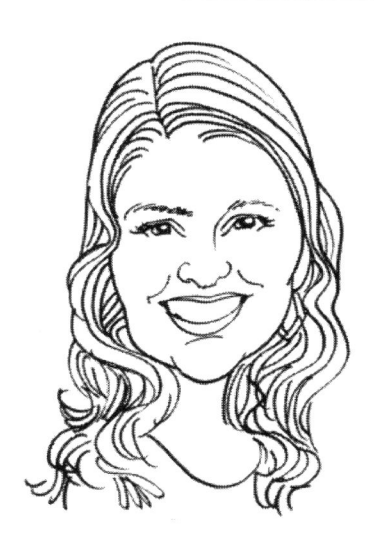

Rebecca Grafton

(@mygirlishwhims)

Rebecca lost 100 lbs. and was featured as a cover girl in people magazine. For her the biggest advice she could give, that helped her along the way was to always start every Monday fresh and back on track. She had tried to "diet" so many times before her most recent attempt and never was successful because, inevitably, she would hit a weekend where she ate crappy and felt like she had derailed all her progress and just decided to give up. She finally learned that no matter how many times he screwed up along the way, every Monday was a fresh start to recommit to her goals and make progress. She made it a habit to always recommit 100% to her goals and healthy lifestyle every Monday, and eventually it became a habit that turned into a lifestyle change. As long as she stayed on track Monday to Friday, she could give herself a little wiggle room to enjoy a few extra treats on the weekend because she knew by Monday she would be back on her game 100%.

She said that KNOWING that she still had some freedom in life to enjoy a hamburger when she wanted one, to drink some extra wine when she felt like it, that all kept her even more committed during the week because she wasn't restricting herself 100% from some of the foods and drinks she really craved. She basically followed the 80/20 rule of healthy living and made sure that every Monday was her start for getting back on track!

> **My Favorite Quote**
>
> "There is no pill, no fad diet, no detox plan, no skinny tea or waist trainer that will lead to you being successful with weight loss. It's only you deciding to take control of your health and fitness and changing your lifestyle that will bring you success."

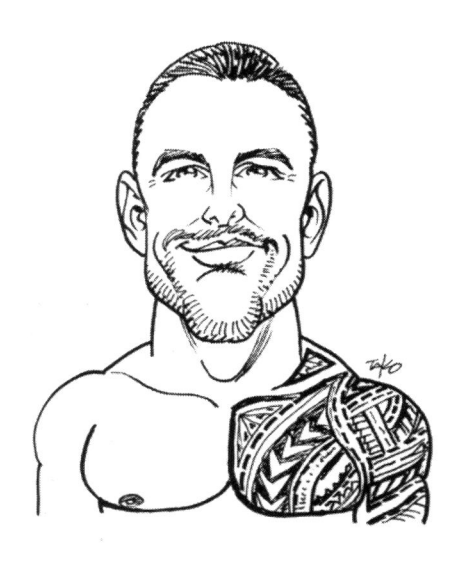

Drew Manning

(@fit2fat2fit)

Drew is the man behind the Fit2Fat2Fit brand. He gained 60 lbs of fat on purpose, eating an unrestricted diet of processed foods to experience what many of his clients were dealing with on a daily basis. After six months of this experiment, he started eating healthy, exercising, and got back into the shape. He called this his Fit to Fat Fit Journey.

Drew is the host of the A&E Hit TV Show Fit to Fat to Fit. He is also a New York Times Best Selling Author for his book FIT2FAT2FIT.

When posed the same question as the others, Drew emphasized that he wants you to make yourself a priority.

He said, "We always give to others, but we put ourselves last. But, you can't pour from an empty cup. It is not selfish to make time for self-care, whether that is going for a walk, meditating, going to the gym, or taking yourself to a movie. You are just as important."

My Favorite Quote

"If we want to grow we must change our mindset and as a byproduct we will then change our whole way of living."

Adry Bella

(@adry_bella)

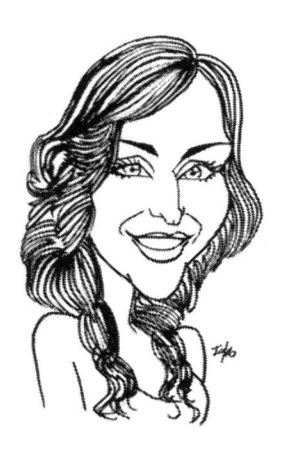

Adry wants us to just get up and do it! Don't even think about it, put on your running shoes your workout clothes and head out the door. Time will pass regardless, it's up to you what you do with it. And I know over until you give up!

> **My Favorite Quote**
>
> "Don't let anyone tell you what you're capable of doing. It's within us all to achieve change, to adapt, to survive, and to strive to be better as each day passes."

By now I hope you are inspired. As you can see from a lot of the advice above, the journey to a healthier life isn't a sprint but a marathon. There will be ups and downs, but as long as you keep at it and never quit, you will eventually reach your goal.

Section 8:

REVIEW, SAMPLE DAY, AND TAKING ACTION

So, you've made it this far. Congratulations!

I've covered a LOT of information on a variety of topics in this book with the goal of helping to empower you to achieve your fat loss and overall health goals through proper nutrition.

This whole "teach a man to fish" methodology is how my trainer Jason went about assisting me on a path to success, and even though I had oftentimes complained to him to "just tell me what to eat, damnit!" Jason stayed the course of empowering me to make my own decisions.

As frustrating as it was at first, in hindsight, I am so thankful that Jason pushed me to learn the basic concepts that I have shared here with you so that I could make my own lifestyle choices instead of relying on someone else to do it for me. Being self-sufficient means I can not only get the results I want, but I can also maintain them for the rest of my life because I am able to adapt and change what, when, and how much I eat to meet the current life situation, no matter how much it changes.

This one basic concept will empower you, the reader, to best be able to eat for your own goals based on your own lifestyle. This is what makes this book so different from the majority of the "diet books" out there. Typically, the base concept found in other nutrition or diet books revolves around telling the reader that there is a "bad guy" food you need to avoid and/or a "superhero" food to focus all your attention on.

As you have hopefully learned here, there is no such thing as a good food or a bad food; rather, the challenge comes when people don't pay attention to their food intake at all. Shifting from a place of confusion and apathy (where most people are with their food intake) to a place where you have a firm grasp on what, when, and how much you need to eat to reach your fat loss goals, means you have been returned to the driver's seat of your own life and are now able to accomplish what you want with your health and fitness goals.

This position of empowerment is yours to wield as you deem appropriate based on what is going on in your life from day to day. Life changes, and that means you need to be able to "roll with the punches" and change your approach to match it. When everything is going smoothly, and your daily routine runs like clockwork, anyone can make their food work for them, but what happens when life throws you a curveball, and you have to change things up? Well, if you were stuck with some other diet plan that required you to eat one way only, you would probably throw your hands up and abandon your focus on eating right as it would become too difficult to bend your lifestyle to meet the demands of your rigid diet plan.

The fact that "shit happens" is the very reason I created The Overeasy System: to empower you through a better understanding of the basic concepts that truly affect change.

My goal was to make this as EASY as possible by wading through all the superdense scientific stuff that usually puts people to sleep and simplifying it into a set of concepts anyone can use to their advantage.

Let's review what we have learned to make sure everything makes sense.

What foods are optimal to help you lose fat and boost energy?

- There is no such thing as a "bad" food, just "bad" quantities.

- Eat whole foods that have been recently "alive" to maximize the thermic effect of food. It takes more energy to break down a whole apple then it takes to break down apple juice, which has already been processed from its original state.

- Minimize "processed" foods as they tend to be very calorie-dense.

- All three macronutrients (carbohydrates, proteins, and fats) have immense value and should be balanced based on your own specific lifestyle.

- The average person's daily food should be composed of approximately 40% protein, 30% carbohydrates, and 30% fat.

- You need carbohydrates (sugar) to fuel your body—just make sure to eat the right amount for your level of activity. The more active you are, the more carbs you'll need to consume.

- A moderate to high amount of protein intake (30-40% of your total calories coming from protein) helps with three key things while in a calorie deficit:

- Protein helps to spare muscle - "Helps maintain your muscle mass during fat loss."

- Protein helps increase satiety - "Makes you feel full."

- Protein has a relatively high TEF - "Takes more energy for your body to process than fats or carbs."

* Coffee and other foods and drinks that contain caffeine can be used to reduce hunger, thereby reducing total food intake.

When should you eat to maximize results?

* Eat as many times per day as works for your own lifestyle and helps to keep you satiated to minimize overeating.

* Intermittent fasting is one method of controlling when you consume food by limiting your food intake to certain times of day.

* Strategically choosing foods throughout the day can help keep you satiated so you won't get cranky or overeat. Either/both of the options below might work for you:

    a. Eat foods higher in healthy fats and protein as they release CCK to aid in early meal termination - "What makes you feel full."

b. Eat leafy greens and other fibrous vegetables as the bulk of the fiber helps to stretch out the stomach, which in turn signals the body to feel full.

- Time the consumption of carbohydrates to fuel your activities such as manual labor or a workout.

    a. Consume complex carbohydrates a couple hours prior to activity to allow for full digestion and absorption.

    b. Consume simple sugars 30 to 60 minutes prior to activity as they digest and absorb very quickly.

    c. Try NOT to do high-intensity exercise in the middle of a fast. Your body needs carbohydrates to optimally perform high-intensity activities, and in the middle of a fast you tend to be very low on blood sugar. Ever get lightheaded during a workout? That's because you're lacking the sugar your brain is looking for to function properly.

How much food should you be consuming to achieve your goals?

- Calories-in versus calories-out is the MOST important factor for achieving your fat loss goals. You can create a calorie deficit by doing one of both of the following:
    - Eat less (calories-in)
    - Move more (calories-out)

- Learn your BMR and put into perspective how much food you should be eating. Want more? Go burn some calories.

- There are three basic ways to track your calories-in:
    - Guesstimate using your hand to gauge approximate calories - This is the least accurate method but the easiest to stick with.
    - Weigh/measure the foods that you eat regularly and try to stick to eating those same foods over and over - Works well for people who don't mind the monotony.
    - Weigh/measure everything, all the time - This is the most effective method for those who are serious

about results, but it can become a little tedious.

- Starting with the "hand method" is a great way to transition from not measuring your food at all.

- Adjust your macronutrient profile to fit your specific lifestyle similar to the following:

Type of person	Protein	Carbs	Fats
Average American	40%	30%	30%
Hungry	30%	30%	40%
Active	30%	40%	30%

- Use a combination of intrinsic and extrinsic accountability to maximize your opportunity for success by doing the following:

    o Track your foods in The Overeasy System app and engage the community to help hold you accountable and motivate you with your successes.

    o Join and engage with The Overeasy System Facebook group to learn what is working for the other group

122

members, find new recipe ideas, and keep up with the latest nutrition information.

- Share your journey on social media.

SAMPLE DAY OF FOOD

So many people ask me to give them an example of what I actually eat on a given day, just so they have an idea of what it looks like, so I figured I would share what my average day looks like here. Due to the moderate level of activity that I have with my running and gym workouts, I use a macronutrient balance of approximately 40% carbohydrates, 30% protein, and 30% fat. I need the extra carbohydrates to fuel my workouts, which is why I increased them above the standard 30%. My total calorie intake on the days I am NOT doing intermittent fasting is about 1,800 kcal.

Meal 1 - Cucumber Tomato Salad with Tuna and Almond Butter with Celery & Carrots

- 4 medium tomatoes, chopped

- 2 cups of lettuce, shredded
- 2 cucumbers, sliced
- 6 oz ahi tuna (RAWWWWW)
- 2 tbsp almond butter
- 2 stalks celery
- 1 cup baby carrots

Meal 2 - BBQ Chicken Breast with Grilled Zucchini

- ½ chicken breast
- ⅓ cup BBQ sauce
- ½ tbsp butter
- ½ tbsp Worcestershire sauce
- ⅓ tsp garlic powder
- 5 zucchini sliced, into spears

Meal 3 - Breakfast Sandwich with Egg, Cheese, and Ham

- 2 English muffins, - toasted
- 2 whole eggs, fried
- 2 oz honey ham, sliced
- 1 oz cheddar cheese, sliced

Nutrition Information:

- Calories - 1758
- Carbs - 175g (39%)
- Fat - 56g (28%)
- Protein - 152g (34%)

This is a pretty average day of food for me as I like to keep things fairly simple.

If I find that I am a little extra hungry, I'll just throw in half an avocado or a handful of almonds, and those extra fats will help keep me feeling full until my next meal.

As you can see, these foods are really simple to prepare, and I like it that way as I don't want to spend too much time preparing things due to my very busy schedule with my job and family life. Just like everything else in The Overeasy System, keeping your food choices as "easy" to make as possible will make them sustainable, and you will stick with it. Once things get too complicated, most people will find excuses to NOT stick with their optimal food intake, and that's why MOST people go through the standard weight loss/weight gain rollercoaster.

Keep it simple and you will be able to eat for a lifetime without having to deprive yourself of the foods you enjoy.

SAMPLE MEAL WHEN BREAKING FAST

As stated above I love breaking a fast with "Breakfast for Dinner." Technically the word breakfast comes from - "Breaking a Fast," but does it have to just be in the morning? You can break your fast at anytime of the day.

I prefer one of the two options below.

Option 1 - Bacon and Eggs

- 3 eggs, fried over-easy
- 2 strips of bacon

- ½ avocado, sliced
- 1 medium tomato, sliced

Nutrition Information:

- Calories - 470
- Carbs - 13g (17%)
- Fat - 32g (41.5%)
- Protein - 32g (41.5%)

Option 2 - Steak and Eggs

- 8 oz new york strip, grilled medium-rare
- 2 eggs, fried over-easy
- ½ avocado, sliced
- 1 medium tomato, sliced

Nutrition Information:

- Calories - 710
- Carbs - 10g (13%)
- Fat - 30g (39%)

- Protein - 37g (48%)

TAKING ACTION

So, you've got all the "tools" you need to be successful with losing that extra body fat, but where do you begin? So many people overwhelm themselves thinking they have to do everything perfect from the get-go because otherwise it's not even worth doing, but that is the opposite of the truth.

The best thing you can do is to take ANY step forward towards your goal instead of freezing in indecision. To help you along the path to success, I will list some simple actions you can take immediately to start getting the results you want. Slowly over time, add in another actionable item and then another, and soon enough you'll be well on your way to losing fat and feeling great.

- Track all your food in the Overeasy System app for five days to better understand your "starting point."

- Join The Overeasy System Facebook group and start engaging with the other members to learn what they are doing to get great fat loss results.

- Pick one to two of your typical processed foods you eat and replace them with whole food choices.

- Add a hard-boiled egg or half an avocado to one or two of your current meals to help you feel fuller for longer.

- Cut back on food intake (fast) starting with a 12-hour period either in the morning (i.e., don't eat breakfast) or the evening (i.e., don't eat dinner) to see how it makes you feel.

It's now time to implement the principles you've learned in this book. We look forward to watching your progress unfold. Please share your journey with us by using #theovereasylife on any social media posts you may make.

If you would like ongoing support, access to professional advice, healthy recipes, and additional bio hacks, you can join The Overeasy Life's Inner Circle and join other like-minded individuals who are trying to live a fitter, healthier, and happier life.

I hope you enjoyed this book. Here's to a less complicated and healthier relationship with food.

Say goodbye to your old life and hello to The Overeasy Life!

BONUS:

30 MINUTE OVEREASY EXERCISE PROGRAM

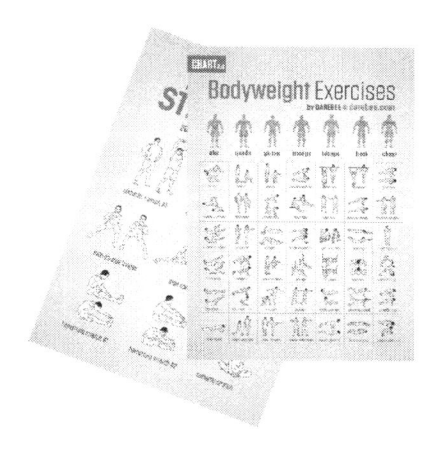

The diagrams above can be found at www.darebee.com

The Overeasy 30 minute exercise program was designed specifically to pack the highest amount of quality exercise into an amount of time that even the busiest corporate executive, stay at home mom, or otherwise time restricted individual can manage to fit into their jam packed day. This easy to do workout will challenge every major muscle group on your body, increasing both strength and muscle tone, while at the same time helping keep you flexible. We kept all of the exercises super simple, focusing on bodyweight movements that require no special equipment and can be done virtually any place, like your own living room, the hotel room during a business trip or even at your local park.

In order to keep this workout as simple as possible, we have split it into 4 basic sections that can be done anywhere, anytime:

1. Warm up - 5 minutes

2. Stretching - 9 minutes

3. Strength - 14 minutes

4. Cool down - 2 minutes

Just so you don't have to worry about getting bored doing the same old exercises over and over, we have included 2 handy exercise charts that include a multitude of exercises for you to pick from. The great thing about these simple to do exercises, is that it doesn't matter what your level of fitness is, they can still really challenge you no matter if this is your first time working out, or if you are an advanced trainee. We have broken the exercises down into 7 body part categories:

1. Abs
2. Quads
3. Glutes
4. Triceps
5. Biceps
6. Back
7. Chest

Every workout will have the same basic structure where you will select one exercise for each body part off of the handy chart we provided you, but instead of doing the same old boring routine each time, you get to use your own artistic license to mix and match exercises so no two workouts will be the same. This allows for nearly endless combinations of exercises in order to help keep your mind stimulated, your body challenged and the results happening. We have made the illustrations for each exercise simple to understand so there are no overly complex movements that will confuse you. This workout is simple, quick and guaranteed to give you results in only 30 minutes a day.

In order for the Overeasy 30 minute exercise program to work for everyone, regardless of experience, we have structured it so all you have to do is modify two key elements to accommodate for your fitness level:

- How frequently you do the workout
    - Beginners: 1-2 days per week
    - Intermediate: 3-4 days per week
    - Advanced: 5-6 days per week
- How fast you do each exercise
    - Beginners: 10-20 repetitions per minute (4-6 seconds per repetition)
    - Intermediate: 20-45 repetitions per minute (1.5-3 seconds per repetition)
    - Advanced: 45-60 repetitions per minute (1-1.5 seconds per repetition)

We recommend starting the Overeasy 30 minute exercise program by performing each exercise relatively slowly with perfect form and only doing the workout 2 times the very first week so that your body can get used to the new workout format and exercises to help minimize any muscle soreness and keep you engaged with the workout. Nobody wants to get so sore they can't move the next day, so take it easy the first couple of workouts and then you can "turn it up" and challenge your body even more.

Here is the basic outline of how the Overeasy 30 minute exercise program will look each time you perform it:

- Warm up - 5 minutes - walking

- Mobility/Stretching - 9 minutes - (see stretch sheet at https://darebee.com/workouts/fighters-stretching.html)
    - Perform each of the 9 stretches, in any order you want, holding each one for 1 minute

- Strength Training - 14 minutes - (see bodyweight exercise sheet at https://darebee.com/muscle-map.html
    - Choose exercise for each body part category
    - Perform a round of all 7 exercises for 1 minute each, executing as many perfect repetitions as possible during the 1 minute
    - Repeat a second round of all exercises for 1 minute each again

- Cool down - 2 minutes - walking

Make sure to keep some water and a towel handy as this workout will make you sweat and get thirsty!

DISCLAIMER You should consult your physician or other health care professional before starting this or any other fitness program to determine if it is right for your needs. This is particularly true if you (or your family) have a history of high blood pressure or heart disease, or if you have ever experienced chest pain when exercising or have experienced chest pain in the past month when not engaged in physical activity, smoke, have high cholesterol, are obese, or have a bone or joint problem that could be made worse by a change in physical activity. Do not start this fitness program if your physician or health care provider advises against it. If you experience faintness, dizziness, pain or shortness of breath at any time while exercising you should stop immediately.

COULD I ASK YOU FOR A FAVOR!

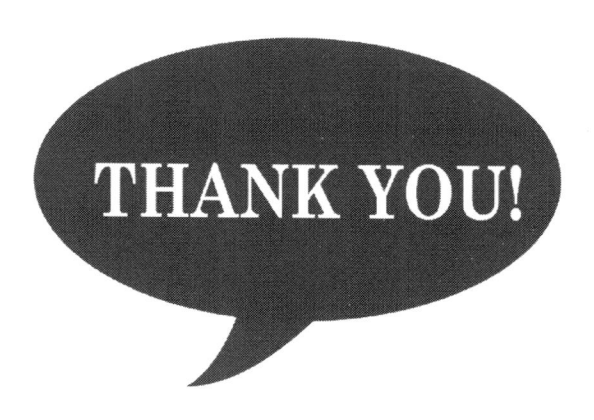

THANK YOU!

Thank You For Reading My Book, and I Would Love To Hear What You Have To Say.

My goal is to help others create a healthier lifestyle and I want to make sure the next version of this book and future books hit the mark.

Please leave me a review on Amazon letting me know what you thought of the book.

To a Fitter, Healthier, and Happier Life!

- Chris Miquel

Made in the USA
San Bernardino, CA
20 June 2018